THE BEGINNER'S GUIDE TO
ACUPRESSURE

DIY STEPS FOR SELF-CARE

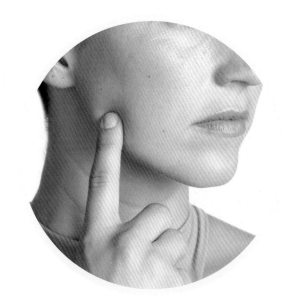

Karin Parramore
LAc, CH

Robert
ROSE

For complete cataloguing information, see page 155.

Disclaimer
This book is a general guide only and should never be a substitute for the skill, knowledge, and experience of a qualified medical professional dealing with the facts, circumstances, and symptoms of a particular case.

     The nutritional, medical, and health information presented in this book is based on the research, training, and professional experience of the author, and is true and complete to the best of her knowledge. However, this book is intended only as an informative guide for those wishing to know more about health and medicine; it is not intended to replace or countermand the advice given by the reader's personal physician. Because each person and situation is unique, the author and the publisher urge the reader to check with a qualified health-care professional before using any procedure where there is a question as to its appropriateness. The author and the publisher are not responsible for any adverse effects or consequences resulting from the use of the information in this book. It is the responsibility of the reader to consult a physician or other qualified health-care professional regarding his or her personal care.

Design and Production: PageWave Graphics Inc.
Editors: Fina Scroppo & Kathleen Fraser
Indexer: Gillian Watts
Model photographer: Kacey Baxter

Additional Images: photographs pages 10, 14, 20, 29, 32 © Getty Images; patterns/illustrations pages 5, 8, 17, 18, 19, 22, 23, 24, 25, 26, 27, 39, 156 © Getty Images; texture pages 6–7, 12–13, 30–31, 106–107 © Getty Images

Published by Robert Rose Inc.
120 Eglinton Avenue East, Suite 800, Toronto, Ontario, Canada M4P 1E2
Tel: (416) 322-6552 Fax: (416) 322-6936
www.robertrose.ca

Printed and bound in China

1 2 3 4 5 6 7 8 9 ESP 32 31 30 29 28 27 26 25 24

THE BEGINNER'S GUIDE TO
ACUPRESSURE

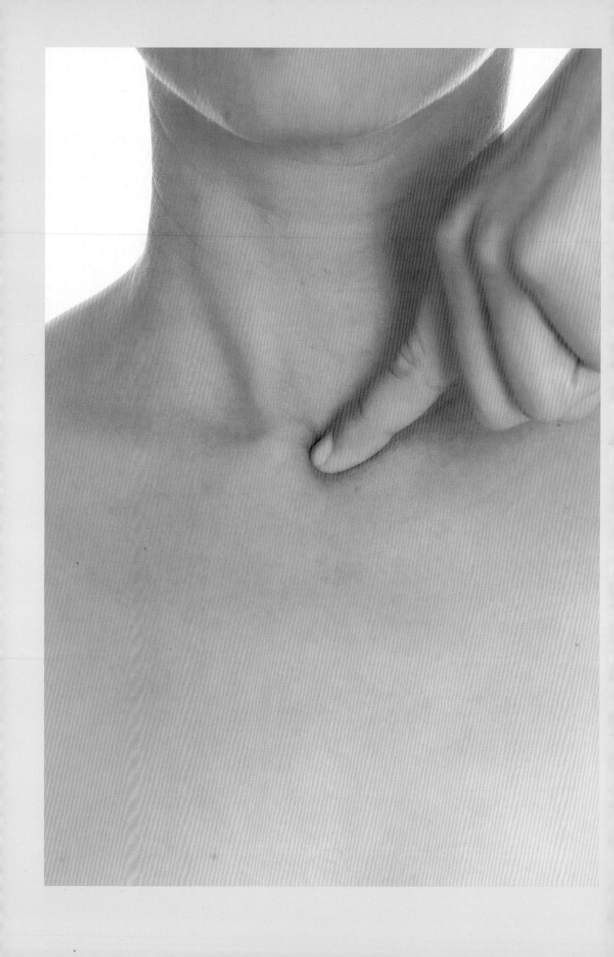

For my
beloved
Minks

CONTENTS

This work is based on thousands of years of accumulated wisdom that still provides healing principles for the modern world. My sincerest thanks to those ancient Chinese medicine scholars who gathered these medical concepts into the classical texts of this system.

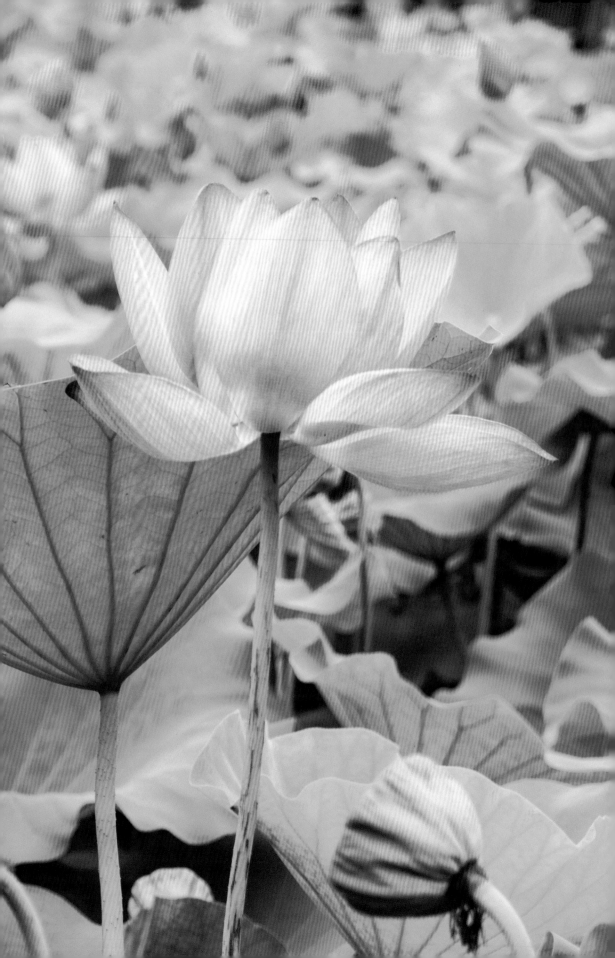

Introduction

This book contains some of the leaves and branches of a vast tree rooted in the concepts of ancient Chinese medicine.

In ancient times, medical scholars looked to the patterns of nature to understand what health should look like. In an age of technological conveniences, many of us have become removed from a direct connection with nature and its rhythms.

When I first encountered this ancient medical system, my teacher was quick to point out that its concepts constitute a system that is just as applicable today, in the modern age, as it has been for many thousands of years. As with any complete system of understanding, these ideas describe a way of knowing that, if valid, should hold true to this day.

In my experience, that is the case. These ideas, this worldview, is so profound and yet also basic that it remains applicable to our current lived experience. Based in natural cycles that have persisted (as far as we know) for all of material existence, these cycles are reliably consistent and help ground us into nature.

This book is intended to be an introduction to acupressure for self-treatment and it is primarily dedicated to reducing symptoms.

By pressing the acupoints as described here, it may be possible to reduce discomfort and increase ease as often as needed in the comfort of your own home. By following the suggestions included here, you can gain increased agency in your own health.

While the book is not intended to cure imbalances, it does aim to offer some relief. It is also my hope that the relief gained by applying the concepts presented here will increase interest in Chinese medicine in general.

For a complete approach to curing root imbalances, I recommend visiting a Chinese medicine practitioner who has the knowledge and training to help you return to a state of balance.

CHAPTER 1

Understanding Chinese Medicine and Its Therapies

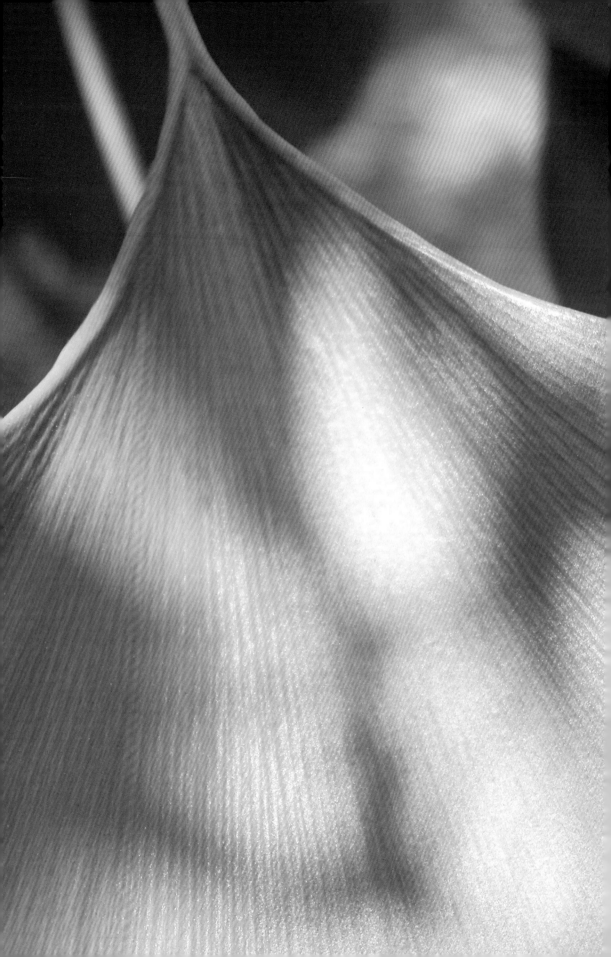

What Is Chinese Medicine?

The therapies you will find in this book refer specifically to an approach to health and healing that arose in China somewhere between 5,000 and 3,000 years ago. The ancient Chinese scholars were prolific recorders of history, and the concepts that underlie this system of healing were preserved in classical texts such as the *YiJing* (also written as *I Ching*), the *Huangdi Neijing (Yellow Emperor's Classic of Medicine)* and the *Shennong Bencao Jing (The Divine Farmer's Classic of Herbal Medicine)*, texts still used by Chinese medicine practitioners today. What these texts demonstrate is that Chinese medicine, over thousands of years, developed into a complete, systematic approach to maintaining health.

At the root of Chinese medicine is a connection to nature. To understand what it means to be a healthy human, the practitioners of old looked to the patterns of nature. Humans (and all living creatures in the material world) were understood to be reflections of larger, more universal patterns that could be "read" through attentive consideration of the world and nature. Seasonal change is a good example. By recognizing the repetitive, cyclic nature of the seasons, we are able to describe a pattern that characterizes that particular time of the year.

The idea is that by taking these universal patterns as models for our lives, we can more easily maintain our health. Not many people would wear a bathing suit outdoors in the winter, for example. We automatically dress warmly without thinking much about it because we know that exposing ourselves to extreme cold will give us a chill, weaken us and, eventually, sap our vitality. While this example may be an obvious one, in truth, all of nature's patterns can inform us about how to stay healthy.

Another key element of Chinese medicine takes into account our surroundings. The health we try to preserve in this tradition is not just our own personal health, but the health of those around us — our community — as well as the environment.

As the ancient scholars observed the world around them for clues, one of the first things they realized was that nothing in nature is static. Rather, the world and its patterns are constantly changing in order to maintain balance. A recognition of this foundational truth helps us adapt in a healthy way.

A BALANCED ACT
The ancient Chinese understood that we are intimately connected to the land we inhabit, and if it is out of balance, we also become out of balance.

QI

In Chinese medicine, all disease starts at the root, as an imbalance of qi. In a nutshell, the basis of Chinese medicine thinking can be defined as assessing imbalances in the flow of qi. These imbalances, if left untreated, will eventually lead to other, more overt problems that we label "diseases."

QI CONNECTION

Qi is a uniquely Chinese concept that is difficult to define. For our purposes here, we will call Qi the vital force that flows through all matter in the universe, including our bodies.

NATURAL PATTERNS DISRUPTED

So, what leads to imbalances in the flow? As mentioned earlier, one of the primary causes is not patterning our lives after the larger universal patterns we observe in the rest of nature. As modern life takes us further and further from these patterns, we see greater and more troubling imbalances.

Chinese medicine can help with imbalances brought about by our disconnection from nature, and the negative influences of modern life, such as pollution. Most important, we can educate the patient about how to reconnect with natural cycles.

Acupuncture and herbs are the primary modalities of Chinese medicine, although bodywork therapies, such as shiatsu and tui na, also play a large role. Chinese medicine practitioners, using acupuncture and acupressure, work to bring fluctuating patterns back into alignment with the patterns that we originally followed naturally.

While acupuncture and acupressure can greatly help, at the root of our treatments we strive to help our patients return to these natural patterns by observing what our patients are eating, how they sleep and, perhaps most important, how they respond to the stress of imbalance.

DISEASE = IMBALANCE

Chinese medicine theory recognizes that most symptoms of disease are the body's attempt to bring itself back into balance. Disease is recognized as a part of oneself, and not an enemy to be conquered.

AT-HOME PRACTICES

Keep in mind that the success of treatment relies on a commitment to self-care — adopting the changes suggested by the practitioner and supporting the treatment with practices such as acupressure at home.

YIN AND YANG

When we say we are "balancing the flow," what we really mean is that we are attempting to correct the interaction between yin and yang. The concept of yin and yang is at the root of Chinese medicine. Yin and yang are complements that work together to maintain balance, as all life needs both matter (the more yin aspect) and energy (the more yang aspect) to function. All the classical texts are basically a long survey of everything as seen through the lens of yin and yang, so let's explore these very important terms.

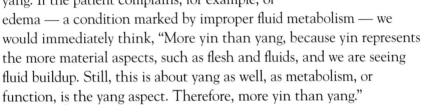

All things in the material world can be defined as containing differing proportions of yin and yang. As doctors, when we take a patient's history, we evaluate if the condition is more yin or yang. If the patient complains, for example, of edema — a condition marked by improper fluid metabolism — we would immediately think, "More yin than yang, because yin represents the more material aspects, such as flesh and fluids, and we are seeing fluid buildup. Still, this is about yang as well, as metabolism, or function, is the yang aspect. Therefore, more yin than yang."

The tendency these days is to see yin and yang as absolutes, to start dividing the world up into this/that: dark is yin, light is yang; male is yang, woman is yin. A better way of stating this would be to say that woman is more yin than man, who is more yang.

In very broad terms, yin is dense matter and yang is diffusive energy. Yin cannot function without yang, and yang cannot be contained without yin to hold it. A living thing in which function and matter are separating is by definition dying.

NO ABSOLUTES
In the material world, nothing is pure yin or pure yang; by definition, any material object is a blending of the two and living matter is impossible without this blending.

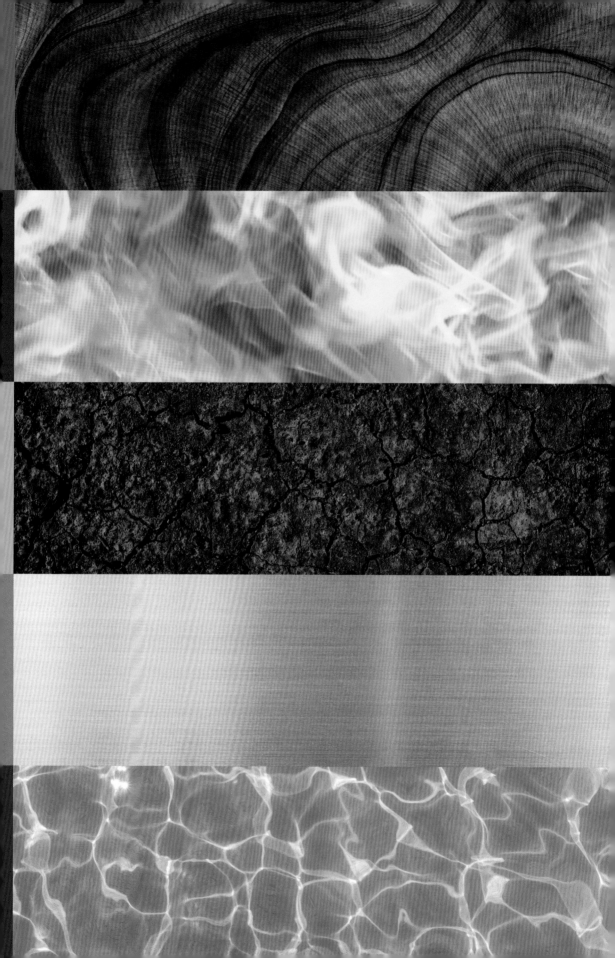

Greater Patterns

When we move beyond the (seeming) duality of yin and yang, it quickly becomes apparent that nature is easily divided into larger patterns as well. Throughout time and across all human experiences, these same ideas have been explored, of course, because they are so basic to life, but each tradition saw the divisions of nature slightly differently. In the European and Western Asian tradition, for example, the four elements were understood as earth, air, fire and water. In China, the idea developed into five elements — wood, fire, earth, metal and water.

THE FIVE ELEMENTS

The five-element system, like the idea of yin and yang, is crucial to Chinese medicine. It is one of the earliest systems for categorizing the material world. Combining the ideas of yin and yang with five elements further refines and clarifies the qualities of yin and yang in specific instances. While the five elements are easy to understand as elements alone, the same characteristics we ascribe to them can be used to understand human physiology and pathology.

Fire, for example, by its very nature is more yang — it is hot, it moves, it is necessary to maintain life. We see the metabolic processes of the body as fire-like. Digestion is understood to be a type of "cooking" within the body that liberates the nutrients in the foods we eat. If we apply the thinking behind yin and yang onto five elements, we see that yang fire implies doubled fire — yang is diffusive energy and enables metabolism — and brings to mind a roaring bonfire that can easily get out of control. This could be at the root of a condition like acid reflux, for example — a digestive fire grown out of control.

The qualities of each element are assigned to all aspects of being alive, both material as well as physiological functions. Wood, for example, is flexible. It moves up primarily, but also out, yet it is also rooted. Anything occurring in nature that moves up from a rooted place will have some association with wood, although the association may not be immediately apparent. Fighting for one's beliefs even in the face of opposition, for example, is a wood quality.

The opposite is also true — inflexibility in any capacity can be viewed as a wood pathology, in other words, a lack of the essential quality of wood. If someone is experiencing inflexibility in their life, working with acupoints on the wood channels can be very effective.

WUXING: THE FIVE ELEMENTS, OR FIVE PHASES

In Chinese medicine, the Five Elements are primarily understood as movements. In fact, the preferred translation of *WuXing* is Five Phases, to indicate the ability of one element or phase to change into another. Therefore, each phase is described as having a particular "gesture" or movement, which can help us decide if we are balanced or imbalanced in a particular area. The gesture is the direction in which the energy, or qi, tends to move. For example, with wood, the gesture in health, or balance, is up and out.

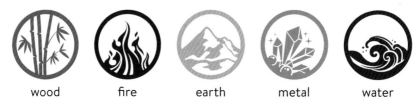

wood   fire   earth   metal   water

It is also important to be aware that each phase can become out of balance in either direction. For example, if healthy wood looks like growth, then wood that is out of balance could be either a lack of growth or uncontrolled growth. This is a very important aspect of the *WuXing*.

To understand better the concepts of *WuXing*, it can help to have some knowledge of the physiologically appropriate attributes or qualities of each of the Five Elements, wood, fire, earth, metal and water. This includes the gestures (or directions of movement) of the elements, both in health and in imbalance, including some common changes or deviations from the normal, which we describe as pathologies.

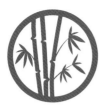

Wood 木

THE GESTURE OF WOOD IN HEALTH: Up and out. Think of a tree — a tree grows up, but the branches spread out. Any physiological activity that mirrors this up-and-out gesture is assigned to wood.

Physiologically appropriate qualities might include:
- Goal-oriented
- Flexible
- Vigorous
- Promotes growth
- Enthusiastic
- Compassionate
- Shows leadership
- Keeps tendons healthy (wood governs all string-like structures in the body, such as tendons, nerves, hair and nails)
- Pushes against gravity (think trees) — wood energy in the body moves blood up through the system
- The person with strong wood traits can be righteously angry. This one is sometimes confusing to folks new to Chinese medicine. The idea is that we harness our anger at injustice for the benefit of those who are being treated unfairly.

THE PATHOLOGICAL GESTURE OF WOOD: Collapsing down and in; in other words, the opposite of the wood gesture in health.

Pathologies might include:
- Inflexibility or overly flexible (both emotionally and physically)
- Narrow-mindedness (overly goal oriented) or inability to set goals
- Stunted or reckless growth
- Inability to rise when help is needed or exhaustion due to agreeing to everything
- Undirected anger or the courage of your convictions
- Blood stagnation, a collapse of the ability to push against gravity
- Tendon weakness

Fire 火

THE GESTURE OF FIRE IN HEALTH: Like wood, fire moves up and out, but it tends to be more expansive, less single-minded or unidirectional. Fire has the ability to rapidly change direction, unlike wood, which tends to move more slowly.

Physiologically appropriate qualities might include:
- The ability to stay warm
- Devoted — imagine the glow when one is gazing upon a loved one
- Enthusiastic bursts of creativity or intuition, like flames dancing in a fire
- Maintains healthy blood flow and vessels (with wood energy)
- Keeps the heart — both the emotional and physiological heart — healthy
- Yang fire is both the central core of our body and the physiological functions that take place at the periphery of the body: maintaining a core temperature is one aspect and keeping the extremities warm is the other.

THE PATHOLOGICAL GESTURE OF FIRE: "Burning out," flying up and away or unable to raise the fire.

Pathologies might include:
- Restlessness or ennui
- Insomnia or inability to stay awake
- Mania followed by depression
- Headaches — fire rising, or edema of the feet: not enough warmth to keep the fluids in the blood
- High blood pressure or chronically low blood pressure

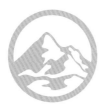

Earth 土

THE GESTURE OF EARTH IN HEALTH: Cycling in and out, which is the ability to go out into the world, experience it and bring it back to center for processing on a personal level — all while maintaining groundedness.

Physiologically appropriate qualities might include:
- Centeredness
- Nurturing
- Generosity
- Maintaining good digestion
- Satisfied with enough for whatever is needed, whoever needs it
- Dynamically stable — able to remain centered in an ever-changing environment; grounded, but in the way a dancer is, or a sailor on a ship

THE PATHOLOGICAL GESTURE OF EARTH: No movement, stuck in the mud, or the feeling we are just "spinning tires."

Pathologies might include:
- Laziness or tendency to be driven solely by other's ideas or desires
- Stuckness (material, emotional, mental, environmental) or inconsistency
- Greediness or carelessness with resources
- Inability to nourish others or being completely self-serving
- Tendency to overeat or inability to eat many things
- Digestive problems

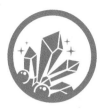

Metal 金

THE GESTURE OF METAL IN HEALTH: Descending — metal is heavy and falls; it can be the sword that cuts away the unnecessary.

Physiologically appropriate qualities might include:
- Healthy elimination
- Healthy respiration
- Uprightness of character
- A tendency to be structured
- Respectfulness
- Willingness to make hard decisions and cut away the unnecessary
- Using ritual as a centering practice and a way to connect to spirit

THE PATHOLOGICAL GESTURE OF METAL: Rigidity or too much descent — freefall.

Pathologies might include:
- Rigidity, both of mind and body
- A tendency to be judgmental, or to be naive
- A tendency to be dogmatic, or too easily swayed
- A tendency to be obsessive or wishy-washy
- A tendency to be a bully or timid
- Weak lung qi
- Constipation

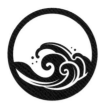

Water 水

THE GESTURE OF WATER IN HEALTH: Go low; completely descended, as in bowing to the awe of the Universe.

Physiologically appropriate qualities might include:
- Humbleness
- Reservedness
- Deeply respectful of the source of life
- Willingness to step aside in favor of another
- Ability to work under another's authority
- Healthy urination and fluid metabolism
- Strong bones; strong, flexible spine

THE PATHOLOGICAL GESTURE OF WATER: Frozen or rigid, inability to descend.

Pathologies might include:
- Excessive or unfounded sense of self-worth or spinelessness
- Tendency to become a recluse, or to be excessively open
- Lack of respect for spiritual matters, or mindless devotion
- Inability to listen to another's opinion, or inability to form one's own opinion
- Stiff-neckedness
- Problems with urination, water metabolism
- Bone diseases, spine problems

Channel Theory

✳

The final key concept of Chinese medicine discussed here is channel theory. Channels are described as the places where the qi, vital energy, flows through the body; that is, the riverways that move vitality to all corners of the body. For acupressure, we use acupuncture points to reach these riverways of vitality.

To speak metaphorically, acupuncture points (acupoints) on the channels can be compared to regions along a river. For example, at junctions of the body with similar features (such as ankles and wrists), the acupoints often have parallel functions, in much the same way that the ports of rivers always occur where the river is wide, deep and calm. Rivers are used to move resources and we want that to occur as seamlessly as possible, at the safest point along the river. It does not make sense to have a port at some rapids, an area defined by fierce and often unpredictable or surprising movement — that region is obviously better for moving swiftly.

HARMONY AND BALANCE

In this chapter, a few of the major concepts of Chinese medicine have been briefly outlined to offer a bit of background to the systems offered elsewhere in this book. The hope is that this short explanation may help readers understand why it works and how this practice can help return us to balance.

Harmony and balance are all-important to Chinese medicine. It is easier to compensate for small changes more often than to try to restore a body that has swung wildly out of balance. Regular use of the techniques described in this book can go a long way to maintaining our native resources and enhancing health.

In the following chapters, we consider further how acupressure interacts with the body and how best to apply it, then we look at some common health conditions that can be treated with acupressure, and then we learn more about the specific acupoints.

CHAPTER 2

Acupressure for Conditions

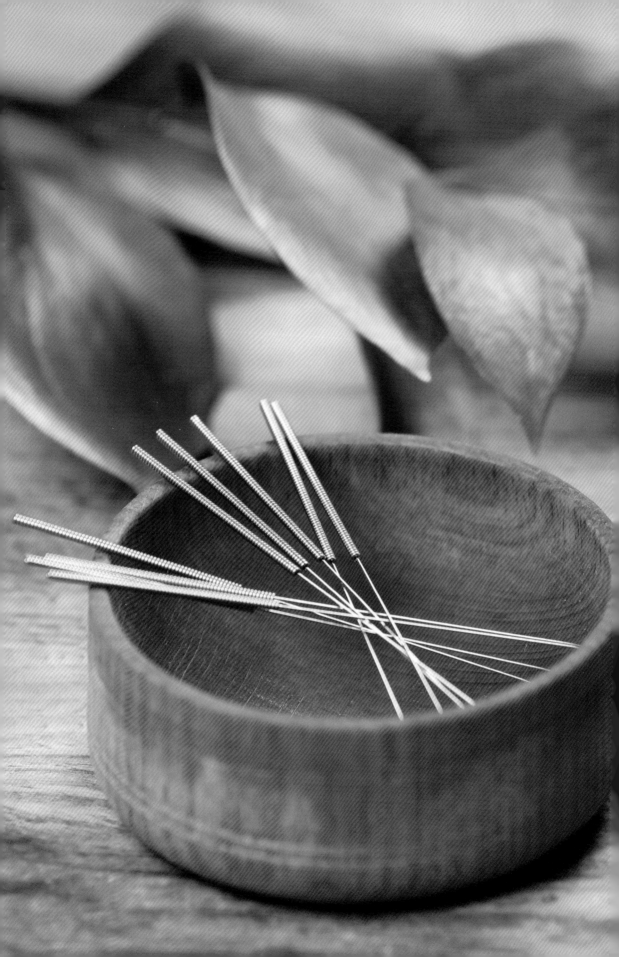

Acupressure vs. Acupuncture

Acupressure is based on acupuncture, a treatment in which filiform (hair-like) needles are inserted into acupuncture points (acupoints) to stimulate a number of different responses. From a purely biomedical perspective, acupuncture is known to stimulate the immune response that occurs any time we insert something foreign into the body. There may be changes in the tissues at the site of the insertion, among other things. Hormonal changes can take place, for example, leading to a sense of calm and relaxation.

From a Chinese medicine perspective, the needle is a conduit for the qi (energy, or life force) in the universe to interact with the qi of both the practitioner and the patient. As described in the chapter on Chinese medicine (see Chapter 1), the patterns of nature guide the patterns within our bodies, and sometimes we need to reconnect with those universal blueprints to maintain a sense of well-being. As an acupuncturist, I can sense changes in the patterns and I work with patients to help smooth the flow of qi. Most times, I am working to remove blockages and encourage qi to return to those places in the body where it is deficient, in order to restore order to the system; in other words, such treatments help the body remember the pattern of health by removing the blocks to health.

In most cases, it takes many years to attain both proficiency at needling and a license to practice acupuncture. For practitioners attempting to work with the root pattern, or source of the imbalance, it makes sense that we would need a great deal of training. The ability to address the symptoms, however, is something everyone should be able to achieve. Reducing discomfort or improving digestion, for example, can greatly improve the quality of life as we work through the process of returning the body to a place of balance.

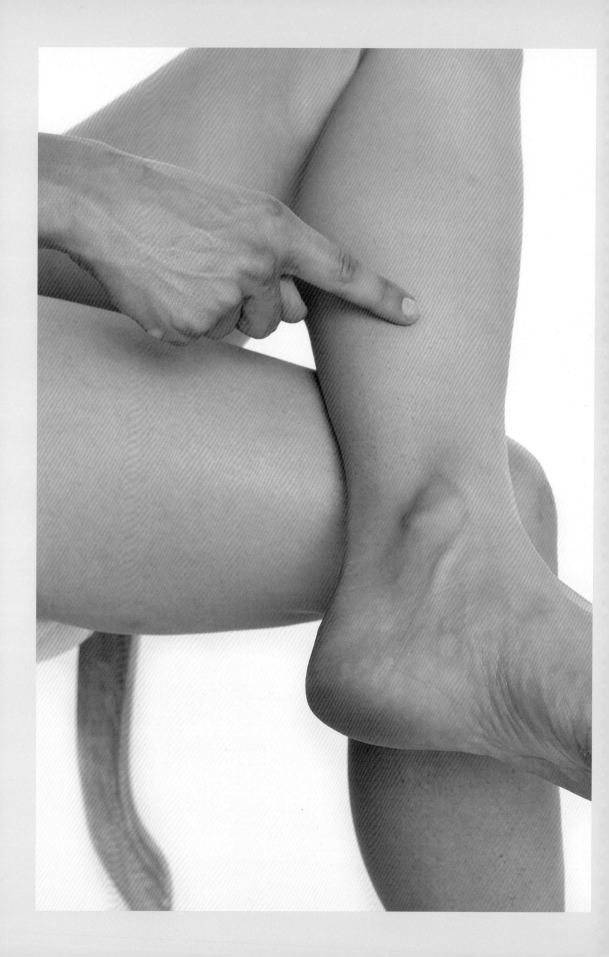

Effective Acupressure Techniques for 34 Common Health Conditions

✳

In this chapter, you will find 34 common health conditions that have been chosen because their symptoms may be effectively reduced by acupressure. Reducing symptoms for any condition can make the recovery process much easier. Even better, these techniques are quite easy to perform on oneself, in the comfort of one's own space.

Acupressure is based on the centuries-old practice of acupuncture. Acupuncture uses acupressure points (acupoints) that are mapped out on the body to interact with the flow of qi (energy, or life force) in the patient. Typically, this is done by inserting extremely fine needles at the acupoint, but in the technique described in this book, the treatment is done through pressure on each point, which is excellent for moving qi. Since most imbalances in the body can be traced to disruptions in the flow of qi, such techniques can be very helpful.

HOW TO USE THESE TECHNIQUES

To use this book effectively, first find the health condition you would like to address. In addition to a synopsis of the condition, there are suggestions for acupressure points (acupoints) that might help. It is important to be very clear about the point location — directions for locations are found in the following pages. Also review the directions for applying pressure and time found on pages 36 and 37.

BEFORE TREATMENT

For the best results, it is important to make time and space for the treatment — try to perform the acupressure when you can focus, in a place where you will not be disturbed or distracted, especially when first learning the technique.

Before you begin pressing, it is important to get a sense of where the points are located on the body. You can learn to do this through sensing tissue changes. This is much easier to experience than most people think. Start by gently palpating — touching mostly with the fingertips — along the lines of the channels to see if you can feel the energy pathway. With practice, you will gain a sense of the course it runs. Next, use the detailed, step-by-step instructions listed throughout this chapter to precisely locate the acupressure points.

APPLYING PRESSURE

Once the point has been confidently located, it is time to apply the pressure. It is not necessary to apply very much pressure. In fact, firm and steady is more important than really deep pressure.

The tissue should not be pressed to the point of frank pain, although it may well be sensitive or uncomfortable (this is often a sign you are on the right track!). If there is an indentation of the tissue that remains for more than 10 seconds after removing your finger, reduce the pressure a bit at the next point. There should *never* be bruising. As mentioned, simply pressing on the acupoint with the intention of smoothing the imbalances can be remarkably effective.

On the other hand, the pressure applied needs to be great enough to easily feel the sensation. Most importantly, pay attention to your body's feedback. Is there an increase in pain or discomfort when you press a point? It may be that the imbalance is resolving, or it may mean you need to lessen the pressure. The more you learn to listen to the feedback, the easier it will become to gauge what your body is telling you.

ACHIEVING BALANCE

Most of the acupoints are bilateral; that is, the points are matched on each side of the body. For most conditions, pressing both acupoints is a good idea — remember, the body is an interdependent system and any influence your treatment exerts will affect the whole body. Balancing will likely happen faster if both sides are equally addressed. If possible, first find and then press both sides at the same time.

If the condition is one-sided, it may be easier to treat the acupoints on the opposite side, especially if a suggested point is close to an area of pain or discomfort. This may seem odd, but because the two sides of the body are basically a mirror image, treating the opposite side will benefit the side with the pain or injury, for a fascinating reason that is beyond the scope of this book.

HOW OFTEN CAN I USE ACUPRESSURE?

The acupoints can be pressed many times throughout the day, as desired. As long as the guidelines regarding pressure are followed, it is difficult, for the most part, to overtreat with acupressure. Again, listen to the feedback from your body. Be sure to also drink a large glass of water following an acupressure treatment.

VARYING TIMES

The length of time to hold each acupoint also depends on personal experience. Some people hold for shorter periods of time but repeat the pressure several times in one treatment. Others suggest holding the point for a set amount of time — for example, 30 seconds to a minute — but these are mostly arbitrary guidelines. We are pressing to smooth the flow of qi; when this starts to happen, we feel it more easily when we learn to listen to our bodies.

When you first begin, start by holding the acupoint for about 30 seconds, then break to see if there is a change — less pain, increased ease in the tissue, for example — before pressing for another 30 seconds. Repeat up to three times in a session.

As always with any treatment, if any unexpected side effects occur, stop pressing. Side effects may include headache, dizziness, nausea or emotional flares. Many people are very responsive to acupressure and do not expect an immediate result even though it's quite normal.

Finally, always try to give yourself at least a minute or two to integrate the changes before leaving the "treatment space." This allows the body to retain the benefits for a longer period of time.

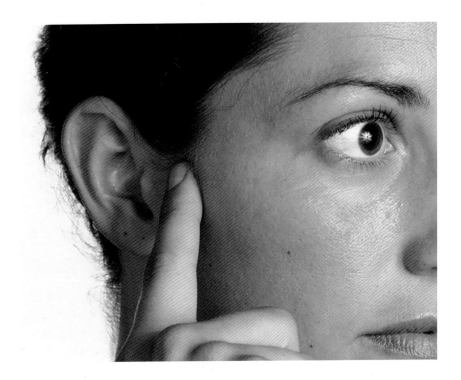

ACCESSING ACUPRESSURE POINTS

It is often necessary to maintain tension in certain parts of the body to access the acupoints on your own. For example, to treat foot points requires bending over, and to access the neck points may require holding the arms up for an extended period, which many people find uncomfortable.

It is important to find the most comfortable position for accessing the points so they can be pressed for an adequate amount of time without leading to discomfort. You will find suggestions for positioning in each acupoint description to help achieve the greatest ease.

SELECTING ACUPRESSURE POINTS

Each acupoint helps specific conditions. Review the conditions described in this chapter as well as the boxes titled "Helps with these conditions" in *Chapter 3: Acupressure Points*, to determine how and when to apply certain acupressure point treatments.

IF YOU NEED HELP

The points described here were chosen first for their function, but accessibility was also a key consideration. Self-treatment requires a person to be able to reach the point easily.

It may be easier, however, to enlist the help of another individual to access some of the points. If someone is assisting, be sure to direct them precisely on where the point is located. Communicate clearly about your responses and give good verbal feedback so the helper does not press too hard, for example.

What I am offering here in this little book is an approach to symptom reduction, to bring comfort and a reduction of suffering. While it is based in some of the classical concepts of Chinese medicine, it is by no means equivalent to the benefits offered by a trained practitioner.

Allergies

Allergies are a hypersensitivity immune response to allergens, defined as substances generally accepted as non-threatening in people without allergies.

The immune system mistakes a non-threatening substance as a threat and mounts an exaggerated response. This usually occurs after a period of hypersensitization, where the allergy sufferer has been exposed to the substance over a long time or in large quantities.

SIGNS AND SYMPTOMS

Typical signs and symptoms include itching, sneezing, runny nose, tearing and congestion. Skin allergy signs include redness, rash or hives, itching and blisters.

NOTE

This treatment is designed to help the allergy sufferer reduce their symptoms and is not intended for people suffering from life-threatening reactions such as anaphylaxis.

Spleen 6 (SP-6 / Sanyinjiao)

This point is located on the lower leg.

1 To locate the point, sit in a chair and cross one ankle over the opposite knee to allow easy access to the lower leg. Locate the inner ankle bone.

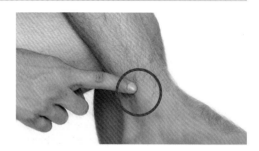

2 Next, place four fingers across the lower leg, with the outer edge of the pinky finger pressing against the ankle bone. Note this line.

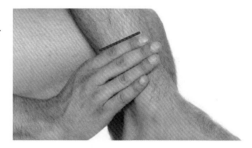

3 Locate the inner back edge of the shinbone (tibia).

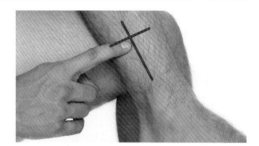

4 Where these two location lines intersect is where you will find the point.

✳ **Warning:** Avoid during pregnancy — can cause contractions.

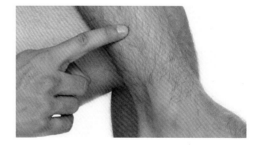

Other Acupressure Points to Consider

After pressing the best acupressure point for this condition, follow with one of these points:

- For allergies with watering eyes, add **BL-2 / Zanzhu** (see Bladder 2, page 129)

- For allergies with excessive watery mucus, add **LI-20 / Yingxiang** (see Large Intestine 20, page 114)

Anxiety Disorder

Anxiety disorder occurs when anxiety starts to interrupt normal behavior.

While conventional medicine describes anxiety as a serious mental disorder, the symptoms usually occur at all levels of being — mental, emotional, physical and spiritual. It may be felt in the body as physical tension, although most sufferers report the mental restlessness as the most distressing symptom.

In Chinese medicine, anxiety is seen as a deficiency of trust in the Dao, or the "way" one's life is unfolding. The inability to feel trust may lead to debilitating uncertainty, creating difficulty with decision making.

SIGNS AND SYMPTOMS

There are many different types of anxiety disorders. Each person may present a totally different set of symptoms. In general, a person with any type will have increased cortisol levels, the body's typical response to stress. There may be increased sweating, agitated movement and signs of panic. Or the opposite signs may appear — retreat, silence and stillness. Either weight loss or weight gain may be seen.

Anxiety can lead to panic attacks, a greatly heightened emotional response that can cause paralyzing fear and erratic behavior, and physical responses such as tachycardia and palpitations. Some anxiety disorders may lead to a withdrawal from activities of daily living, often due to fear of the panic attack itself, which can occur with no apparent trigger when the sufferer is outside of their comfort zone. Agoraphobia (fear of the outside) may arise as well.

> **NOTE**
> Both hyperthyroidism and adrenal tumor may cause anxiety.

Pericardium 6 (PC-6 / Neiguan)

This point is located on the inner forearm close to the wrist.

1 To locate the point, rest the arm on a comfortable surface, palm side facing up.

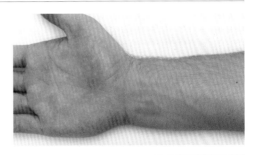

2 Place two middle fingers from your left hand on your right forearm so that the middle finger lays facedown over the wrist crease. Where the index finger falls is the horizontal location line. Note the line and remove your left hand from your forearm.

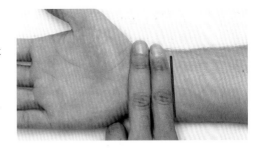

3 Next, locate the tendon in the center of the forearm by bending your hand at the wrist so that the palm is moving up, toward the elbow.

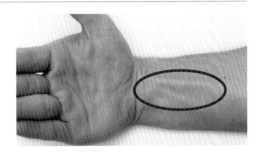

4 Where the horizontal location line intersects the tendon is where you will find the point. Bring your hand back down before pressing the point.

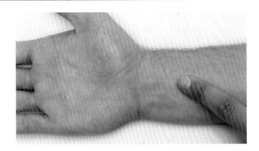

Other Acupressure Points to Consider

After pressing the best acupressure point for this condition, follow with one of these points:

- For non-specific anxiety, add **Yintang** (see page 152)

- For social anxiety, add **Ht-7 / Shenmen** (see Heart 7, page 125)

Arthritis

Arthritis is a degenerative condition of the joints.

Osteoarthritis is usually a result of wear and tear and is more commonly found in people over 60. If the condition develops in a younger person, it usually has a specific etiology, such as injury. The symptoms usually develop and worsen over time. The tendons, cartilage and bursae deteriorate until the bone is no longer cushioned but is working against bone.

SIGNS AND SYMPTOMS

Osteoarthritis is characterized by increased stiffness and pain and decreased range of motion. As the condition progresses, the connective tissue becomes nonfunctional and shrinks, while the bones enlarge, causing the joints to deform. Women are more likely to develop this condition than men.

NOTE

Arthritis with an acute onset may indicate an infectious process such as Lyme disease or a gonococcal infection.

Small Intestine 3 (SI-3 / Houxi)

This point is located on the lateral (outer) side of the hand.

1 To locate the point, slide the tip of the index finger along the pinky finger toward the wrist.

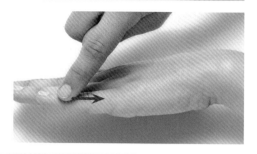

2 Slide the tip of the finger over the first joint of the pinky finger and onto a depression on the outer side of the hand.

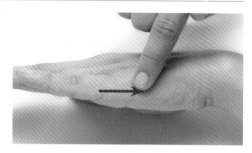

3 The depression lies between the pad on the outer edge of the palm (the hypothenar eminence) and the long bone along the side of the hand (the metacarpal of the pinky finger).

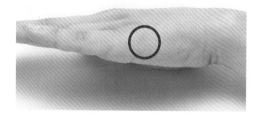

4 Where the finger lands on the center of this depression is where you will find the point.

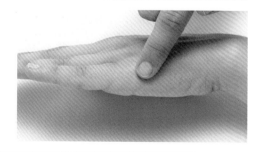

Other Acupressure Points to Consider

After pressing the best acupressure point for this condition, follow with one of these points:

- For arthritis in joints of the upper body, add **SI-1 / Shaoze** (see Small Intestine 1, page 126)

- For arthritis of the lower body, or for stiffness and pain from osteoarthritis, add **GB-34 / Yanglingquan** (see Gallbladder 34, page 142)

Bloating

Bloating is typically due to retention of gas in the gastrointestinal tract, but it can also be caused by retained fluids or stool.

Bloating may be caused by overeating, eating foods that are difficult to digest, food sensitivities or allergies, constipation or eating while experiencing stress. Many digestive disorders, such as inflammatory bowel disease (IBD) or celiac disease, may also present with bloating. In babies, the condition of bloating is called colic.

SIGNS AND SYMPTOMS

The most common symptom is swelling, but it is often accompanied by discomfort or pain in the gut. There is an increased likelihood of flatulence, especially if food sensitivities are the cause. There may be decreased appetite, nausea and vomiting. Irritability is common.

NOTE

Intestinal obstruction can result in bloating, and may be an emergency situation. Bloating may also be a symptom of many diseases, including a number of different kinds of cancer and liver disease. If the bloating is from an undiagnosed cause or worsens suddenly, see a doctor.

ABDOMINAL MASSAGE

Lie on your left side. Starting at the lower right quadrant (near the top of the right hip bone), slowly and gently massage around the abdomen in small circular motions, moving up the right side, across under the ribs and down the left side until the discomfort is relieved.

Stomach 36 (ST-36 / Zusanli)

This point is located on the lower leg, one hand's width down from the knee crease, and one thumb's width lateral (to the right of) the shinbone.

1 To locate the point, extend your leg while seated on a bed or floor.

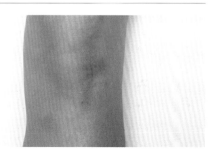

2 Place your left hand on your right lower leg (shin) so that the index finger bumps up against the kneecap (patella). Where your pinky finger falls is the horizontal location line where you will find the point. Note the line and remove your left hand from your shin.

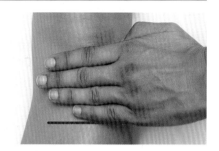

3 Next, place your right thumb vertically next to the shinbone so that the left edge of your thumb presses against the shinbone, and the widest part of your thumb falls across the horizontal line you just located. The right side of your thumb defines the vertical location line. Note this line.

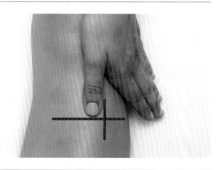

4 Where these two location lines intersect is where you will find the point.

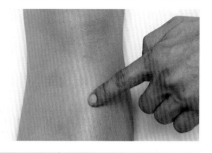

Other Acupressure Points to Consider

After pressing the best acupressure point for this condition, follow with one of these points:

- For bloating with pain, add **CV-12 / Zhongwan** (see Conception Vessel 12, page 148)

- For bloating with diarrhea, add **ST-25 / Tianshu** (see Stomach 25, page 118)

Bowel Incontinence

With this condition, patients experience a decreased control over bowel movements.

It may be temporary, as in the case of food poisoning, when the body's natural defenses are trying to clear toxins as quickly as possible. It may occur as a result of nerve damage following childbirth or surgery, or because of chronic disease, such as diabetes. Increased age also leads to less muscle tone; anal leakage is common in the elderly. Men who have prostate cancer often have a greater likelihood of bowel incontinence, either due to structural change or treatment.

Digestive disorders like ulcerative colitis or irritable bowel disease (IBD) can have bowel incontinence as a symptom.

SIGNS AND SYMPTOMS

Loss of bowel control is the main sign. There may be pain or cramping if it is a result of food poisoning, or it may be accompanied by blood if the cause is a gastrointestinal disorder. If the condition occurs because of age, the leakage may be a small amount, while other causes may result in explosive diarrhea.

NOTE

If symptoms get worse or if the volume of stool loss goes up dramatically, see a doctor.

Conception Vessel 4 (CV-4 / Guanyuan)

This point is located on the lower abdomen.

1 To locate the point, stand in front of a mirror. Expose the lower abdomen.

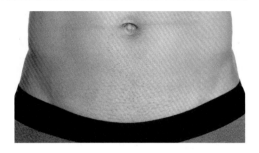

2 Locate the belly button (umbilicus). Place a finger on it.

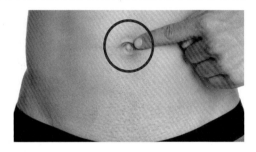

3 Next, slide the finger down about four fingers' width.

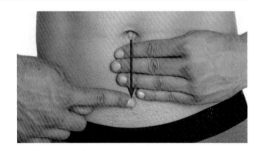

4 Where the finger lands on the swell of tissue just under the belly button is where you will find the point.

✳ **Warning:** Avoid during pregnancy — may cause too much pressure on the baby.

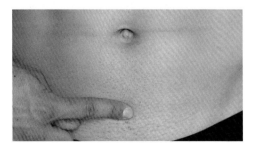

Other Acupressure Points to Consider

After pressing the best acupressure point for this condition, follow with one of these points:

- For bowel incontinence after a long illness, add **SP-6 / Sanyinjiao** (see Spleen 6, page 122)

- For bowel incontinence due to anal prolapse, add **GV-20 / Baihui** (see Governing Vessel 20, page 151)

Carpal Tunnel Syndrome

The term refers to a collection of symptoms resulting from pressure on the median nerve, the primary nerve serving the hand and fingers.

With this condition, the median nerve becomes trapped in the carpal tunnel, a small gap created by the transverse carpal ligament and the bones of the wrist. In addition to the nerve, the tendons responsible for moving the fingers pass through this small space. If inflammation of the tissues occurs as a result of overuse (repetitive movements such as typing, for example), the nerve is caught between the swollen tissue and the bones, resulting in diminished function.

SIGNS AND SYMPTOMS

In addition to diminished function, carpal tunnel syndrome usually results in tingling, numbness and fatigue of the hand. There is often associated pain — often sharp and stabbing — and there may be an electric sensation. Pain may radiate to other areas, commonly up the arm toward the elbow.

Proper ergonomics when performing repetitive tasks is crucial. Many computer keyboards are designed to keep the hands in a more natural position when typing, while pads can help support the wrists.

The condition may spontaneously reverse and normal function return with no treatment at all; however, this is not usual. The conventional treatment is surgery, and braces may be helpful in some cases. Oral corticosteroids are also regularly prescribed.

> **NOTE**
>
> Carpal tunnel syndrome may be associated with other diseases such as hypothyroidism and diabetes, and pregnancy can exacerbate the condition.

Pericardium 7 (PC-7 / Daling)

This point is located on the inner forearm, on the wrist crease.

1 To locate the point, rest the hand on a comfortable surface, palm side facing up. Locate the wrist crease by slightly bending the hand up. Relax the hand.

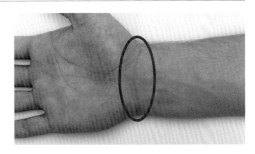

2 Next, locate the tendon at the center of the wrist.

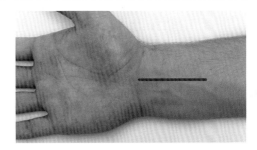

3 Tensing all fingers will engage the tendon, making it easier to find.

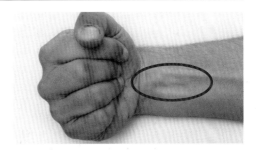

4 Where the wrist crease and the tendon intersect is where you will find the point.

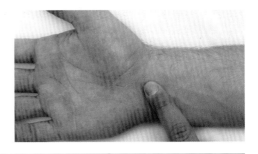

Other Acupressure Points to Consider

After pressing the best acupressure point for this condition, follow with one of these points:

- For carpal tunnel syndrome with heat, add **LU-11 / Shaoshang** (see Lung 11, page 110)

- For carpal tunnel syndrome with cold, use **Ht-7 / Shenmen** (see Heart 7, page 125)

Common Cold

The common cold is viral infection resulting in a typical (common) set of symptoms.

The main culprits are respiratory syncytial virus, rotavirus, rhinovirus and coronavirus. These viruses can survive on surfaces outside of the body long enough to infect others — most people catch a cold when they come in contact with the causative agent after someone sneezes or coughs. Doorknobs and light switches, for example, are surfaces we regularly touch without thinking.

Those most at risk include babies and children, the elderly and the immunocompromised. If the immune system is weakened or suppressed, a simple common cold can be a serious problem.

SIGNS AND SYMPTOMS

Stiff neck, fatigue, a feeling of general malaise, headache, sore throat, fever and chills, sneezing, coughing, runny nose and other symptoms can manifest with the common cold.

OTHER TREATMENTS
• Garlic and onion soup, preferably made with a bone broth base

Lung 7 (LU-7 / Lieque)

This point is located on the crest of the forearm, very close to the wrist.

1 To locate the point, rest the hand on a comfortable surface, palm side facing up. Locate the wrist crease by slightly bending the hand up. Relax the hand.

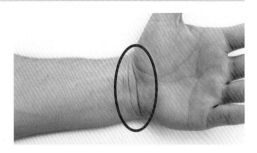

2 With your other hand, lay the three middle fingers horizontally along the crease, with the fourth (ring) finger positioned on the crease itself.

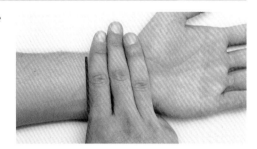

3 Next, roll the tip of the index finger up and over the radius bone, the bone on the thumb side of the forearm.

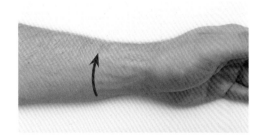

4 Where the tip of the finger lands on the radius bone is where you will find the point.

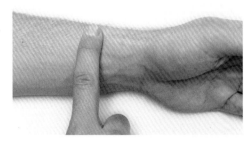

Other Acupressure Points to Consider

After pressing the best acupressure point for this condition, follow with one of these points:

- For cold with fever, add **LI-4 / Hegu** (see Large Intestine 4, page 111)
- For cold with fatigue, add **SP-6 / Sanyinjiao** (see Spleen 6, page 122)
- For cold with alternating chills and fever, add **GB-43 / Xiaxi** (see Gallbladder 43, page 143)

Constipation

While constipation is commonly understood to be slow or difficult bowel movements, medically it is defined as fewer than one complete bowel movement a day.

Constipation has many causes. Dehydration and lack of fiber can lead to small, dry stools, a situation more easily addressed by changes in diet. Lack of tone in the bowel, medications, bowel surgery, restricted exercise, dietary sensitivities and age can all result in slower transit time.

SIGNS AND SYMPTOMS

The two most common forms of constipation are a very slow transit time with normal stool or regular movements but with dry, small, pebbly stools. In addition to a slower bowel movement, it may feel as though the bowel movement is incomplete. Constipation can lead to a need to strain — a tendency that usually leads to other problems, such as hemorrhoids or rectal bleeding. There is often pain, especially with dry stool.

NOTE

If the symptoms continue for more than a week, or if there is a complete lack of bowel movement, it may indicate a blockage in the bowel — contact a doctor as soon as possible.

CAUTION: Be wary of over-the-counter laxatives — using them for extended periods can make the problem worse.

OTHER TREATMENTS
- Ensure adequate fiber, water and oil in the diet. If the constipation is due to lack of motility rather than dehydration, consider abdominal massage to help the muscles of digestion do their job

Stomach 25 (ST-25 / Tianshu)

This point is located on the abdomen, at the level of the belly button, or umbilicus.

1. To locate the point, lie down and expose the lower abdomen. Locate the belly button. Place three fingers vertically (fingertips pointing down) against the lower abdomen, measured from the belly button, so that the edge of the index finger is against the outer edge of the belly button.

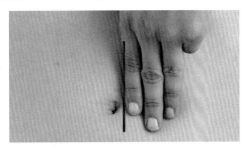

2. Where the third finger ends up on the abdomen, mark an imaginary vertical line. Slide the tip of the index finger along an imaginary horizontal line to the point where the two lines intersect. Where there is a slight depression you will find the point. Note the point.

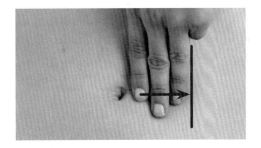

3. Next, locate the point on the opposite side of the abdomen.

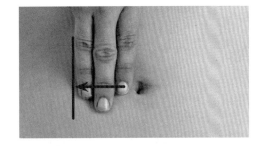

4. Using the index fingers, press both points at the same time.

✳ **Warning:** Avoid during pregnancy — can cause contractions.

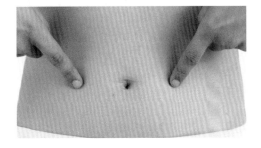

Other Acupressure Points to Consider

After pressing the best acupressure point for this condition, follow with one of these points:

- For constipation with feeling of incompletion, add **ST-36 / Zusanli** (see Stomach 36, page 119) followed by **KI-3 / Taixi** (see Kidney 3, page 133)

Cough

Cough is not actually a condition but a symptom. It is the body's attempt to remove something foreign from the lungs and is characterized by a forceful expulsion of air against the resistance of the diaphragm, which is why prolonged coughing can lead to abdominal pain.

Cough could be a response to an irritant lodged in the airways. It may also occur as the body attempts to expel phlegm-containing infectious agents during a cold or flu. Certain chronic respiratory conditions, such as asthma or bronchitis, are usually associated with cough. Allergies can also bring on cough.

SIGNS AND SYMPTOMS

There are many different types of cough. Those associated with infectious agents usually produce yellow or green phlegm. Allergic cough is characterized by copious, thin to watery clear phlegm. If the cough is extreme, the phlegm may be pink as tiny capillaries in the lungs burst under increased pressure. An unproductive (dry) cough often occurs at the end of a cold or respiratory infection.

Any persistent or exhausting cough, especially in the very young or the elderly, should be examined by a doctor.

NOTE

If there are urinary or bowel changes, or there is a sudden sharp pain in the chest and it does not change, see a doctor.

OTHER TREATMENTS
• For a cough due to allergies, see page 40

Conception Vessel 22 (CV-22 / Tiantu)

This point is located on the lower neck.

1 To locate the point, stand in front of a mirror.

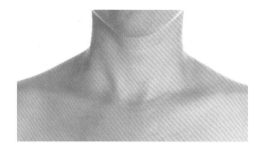

2 Slide the index finger over the breastbone (sternum) to find the notch in the center of the top of this bone.

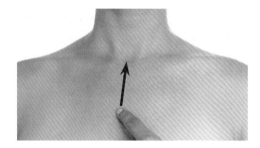

3 The point is actually located behind the bone, so it is best pressed by gently rolling the finger up and over the breastbone, into the hollow behind it.

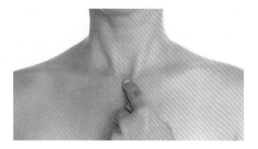

4 Be careful not to apply pressure to the Adam's apple (hyoid bone), which is located just above this point.

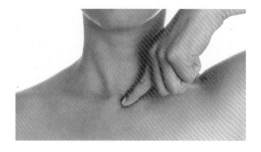

Other Acupressure Points to Consider

After pressing the best acupressure point for this condition, follow with one of these points:

- For cough with sticky yellow mucus, add **LU-7 / Lieque** (see Lung 7, page 108)

- For cough with pain in the chest, add **LR-3 / Taichong** (see Liver 3, page 144)

Depression

Depression is considered a mental emotional disorder wherein the symptoms overwhelm the capacity to live a typical life. How this manifests will be different for each patient.

The incidence of depression is on the rise, as many find it difficult to navigate a rapidly changing world. There is often a triggering event, such as an unexpected change of circumstances (divorce, death, a troubling medical diagnosis), or it may develop idiopathically (no known cause). Recent treatment plans have helped patients manage the disease so it is no longer so debilitating.

One type of depression, seasonal affective disorder (SAD), is precipitated by a lack of sunlight. Diet plays a huge role in depression — one study links increased sugar consumption with increased depression and a greater consumption of fruit and vegetables with decreased symptoms.

Some medications, including many that treat depression, caution that depression may be a side effect.

SIGNS AND SYMPTOMS

Most commonly, those with depression experience exhaustion, lack of energy for daily activities and no inclination to engage with society and life in general. There are often physical symptoms as well, such as decreased or increased appetite, digestive changes and body weakness or heaviness, among others.

NOTE

Depression can manifest as mild to extreme. People who experience extreme symptoms may be considered at risk of committing suicide. If a person is experiencing extreme symptoms, it is very important that they seek professional help. The suggestions here may help manage milder symptoms.

Heart 7 (Ht-7 / Shenmen)

This point is located on the forearm, at the wrist crease.

1 To locate the point, rest the hand on a comfortable surface, palm side facing up.

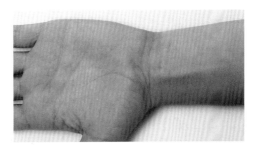

2 Locate the wrist crease by slightly bending the hand up. Relax the hand.

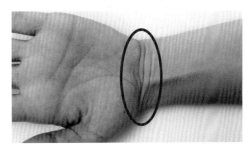

3 Next, slide the tip of the index finger along the wrist crease toward the small bone of the wrist located directly beneath the pinky finger.

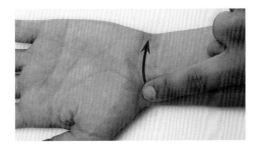

4 Where the wrist crease and the wrist bone meet is where you will find the point.

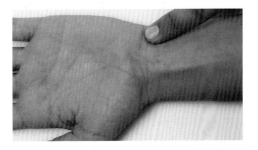

Other Acupressure Points to Consider

After pressing the best acupressure point for this condition, follow with one of these points:

- For depression with a crisis of faith or spirit, add **KI-9 / Zhubin** (see Kidney 9, page 135)

- For depression due to exhaustion, add **ST-40 / Fenglong** (see Stomach 40, page 120)

Diarrhea

While diarrhea is commonly understood as stool that is loose to watery, medically speaking, diarrhea is defined as an increase in bowel movements that have less consistency, or regular frequency but looser consistency.

Diarrhea is a symptom of many acute and chronic diseases. Bacterial and viral infections are the most common cause of acute diarrhea.

Diarrhea is the body's natural response to poisoning, from alcohol or over-medicating, for example, as an attempt to purge the irritant.

SIGNS AND SYMPTOMS

The main sign is an increased number of bowel movements; specifically, more than three a day. Bowel movements may be loose to watery or foamy. Diarrhea is often accompanied by cramping or other gastrointestinal (GI) pain. There may also be a sensation of heat, dizziness, nausea or sweating. Short-term weakness often occurs with acute diarrhea, whereas a chronic case can be debilitating.

NOTES

If the stool contains mucus or blood, it may a sign of a more serious condition.

Stay hydrated while diarrhea continues! Contact a physician if diarrhea is ongoing for more than 48 hours (sooner in small children, the elderly or convalescing patients) because dehydration is a very serious consequence and intravenous fluids may be necessary.

Conception Vessel 12 (CV-12 / Zhongwan)

This point is located on the abdomen.

1 To locate the point, stand in front of a mirror. Expose the abdomen.

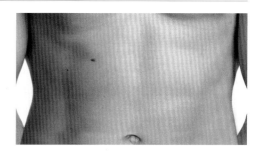

2 Slide the index finger to locate the bottom of the xiphoid process, the lower end of the breastbone (sternum). If the xiphoid itself cannot be located, find the point where the ribs join the low end of the breastbone as a reference point.

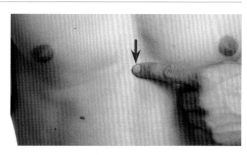

3 Next, locate the belly button (umbilicus).

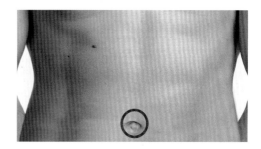

4 The midway point between these two structures, about six fingers' width down from the sternum or up from the belly button, is where you will find the point.

✳ **Warning:** Avoid during pregnancy — may cause too much pressure on the baby.

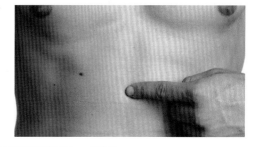

Other Acupressure Points to Consider

After pressing the best acupressure point for this condition, follow with one of these points:

- For diarrhea with cold sensation, add **SP-8 / Diji** (see Spleen 8, page 123)

- For diarrhea with colitis, add **ST-25 / Tianshu** (see Stomach 25, page 118)

Eczema (Atopic Dermatitis)

Atopic dermatitis (eczema) is an inflammatory condition of the skin. The latest findings suggest it is an autoimmune condition.

Two proteins have been determined to act as antigens, and drugs blocking the signaling of these proteins have been found to reduce symptoms.

The hygiene hypothesis suggests that children raised in hyper-sterilized homes are more likely to develop both eczema and asthma, two conditions commonly seen together. When a child encounters a trigger, a flare-up occurs. Unfortunately, nearly anything can act as a trigger, but more recently the main culprits have been soap, shampoo, detergents and synthetic and chemical additives in topical skin-care products. Baby eczema is very common — switching laundry detergent to something more natural and gentle often resolves the issue.

SIGNS AND SYMPTOMS

Each case of eczema is distinctive in presentation, but generally there will be an itchy red raised rash. Tiny blisters often appear; as they develop they may ooze, a development that frequently leads to cracked skin. If the condition continues, the cracks may bleed and scab. The hardened tissue then easily reopens, making it difficult to heal.

NOTE

Excessive use of topical steroids for eczema is believed to drive the condition deeper into the system, often manifesting later as asthma. Avoid topical steroids if at all possible.

Large Intestine 11 (LI-11 / Quchi)

This point is located on the forearm, very close to the elbow.

1 To locate the point, bend the arm 90 degrees.

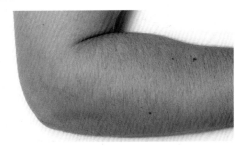

2 With the tip of the index finger from the opposite hand, locate the outermost end of the elbow crease.

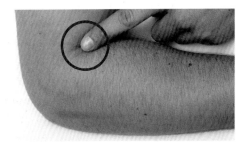

3 Next, slide the finger (away from the body) three fingers' width toward the elbow bone to locate the bony prominence (olecranon process) of the elbow, closest to the elbow crease.

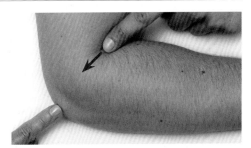

4 Where the finger lands on the midpoint between the elbow crease and the olecranon process is where you will find the point.

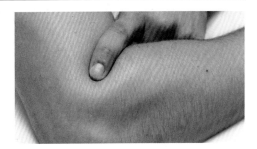

Other Acupressure Points to Consider

After pressing the best acupressure point for this condition, follow with one of these points:

- For atopic dermatitis with red, hot skin, add **LU-7 / Lieque** (see Lung 7, page 108)

- For dry, cracked, bleeding eczema, add **SP-10 / Xuehai** (see Spleen 10, page 124)

Frozen Shoulder (Adhesive Capsulitis)

Adhesive capsulitis, commonly known as frozen shoulder, is a condition that causes pain in the shoulder, followed by stiffness.

Adhesions form that cause the muscles to stick to each other, dramatically reducing the ability of the muscles to function. The muscle bodies can tear apart with activity, and this tearing leads to the creation of scar tissue, further limiting movement and function.

Frozen shoulder often arises very quickly, in some cases overnight, although it is usually a result of an injury or repetitive movement and poor ergonomics. The after-effects of shoulder surgery (with its associated scar tissue) may develop into adhesive capsulitis, which is why it is so important to exercise the healing joint as soon as comfortably possible. Frozen shoulder will often self-resolve after a period of time; the average healing time is 9 to 18 months.

SIGNS AND SYMPTOMS

The condition starts with severe pain during the "freezing" stage, which fades after a short time to extreme stiffness and radically reduced range of motion. There is often crepitus ("creaking") in the joint. Muscle weakness, combined with the poor range of motion, can effectively take the affected arm out of commission.

Post-menopausal women are most likely to develop frozen shoulder.

OTHER TREATMENTS
- Add a warm, moist compress or poultice and heating pad to help with stiffness and pain

Large Intestine 15 (Jianyu)

This point is located on the front of the shoulder.

1 To locate the point, stand in front of a mirror. Bend the arm 90 degrees and raise the elbow until it is level with the shoulder.

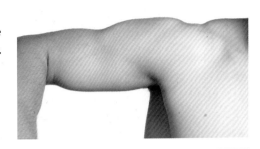

2 This will cause two depressions to appear next to each other at the top of the shoulder. If they are not obvious, palpate for them just above the deltoid muscle at the top of the arm.

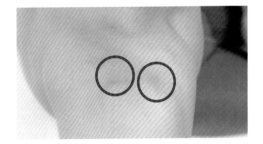

3 Next, use the index finger from the opposite hand to find the depression that is in the front.

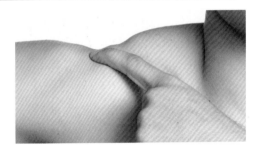

4 Where the finger lands on the depression closest to the chest is where you will find the point. Be sure to relax the arm before pressing the point.

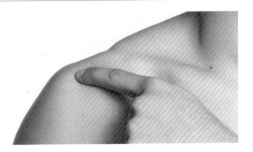

Other Acupressure Points to Consider

After pressing the best acupressure point for this condition, follow with one of these points:

- For anterior frozen shoulder with pain, add **LU-7 / Lieque** (see Lung 7, page 108)

- For posterior frozen shoulder with pain, add **TW-14 / Jianliao** (see Triple Warmer 14, page 139)

Headache

The different types of headache define areas where the pain is experienced (such as frontal or occipital) or point to the different causes (tension, for example).

Frontal headaches are felt mostly in the forehead. Temporal headaches can occur anywhere along the side of the head. Occipital headaches are felt along the occiput, the bony ridge at the back of the head. Tension headaches usually occur in a band around the head, and vertex headaches are felt at the top of the head. Cluster headaches appear in the same spot again and again, but usually each episode does not last long. They are one-sided and often occur around or behind the eye.

Dehydration may also be a cause. Lack of sleep, diet and dietary change — such as reducing sugar or caffeine — stress and medications have all been implicated in the onset of headache.

SIGNS AND SYMPTOMS

Pain is of course the main symptom, but other symptoms may vary and include irritability, inability to focus, dizziness (especially with migraine headaches), nausea and vomiting. Some headaches are associated with a different set of symptoms with each presentation; specifically, migraine sufferers may experience extreme light sensitivity, visual changes and little pain, or the pain may be so severe that they retreat from life for a few days. Typically, the neck and shoulders are involved.

NOTE

Headaches can be a sign of a more serious condition. If they occur with increasing frequency or intensity, visit your doctor. If vision changes occur, it may be an emergency situation. Migraine headaches are unique and should be diagnosed by a doctor. The sudden onset of an excruciating headache is probably an emergency situation.

Large Intestine 4 (LI-4 / Hegu)

This point is located on the back side of the hand, near the base of the thumb.

1 To locate the point, move the thumb toward the index finger until the two are pressed together. This will cause a fleshy mound of skin to bunch up on the back of the hand, between the index finger and thumb.

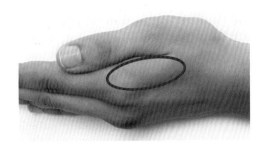

2 Find the highest point at the center of this mound.

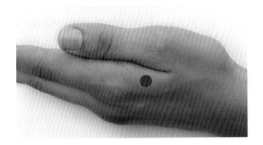

3 Where the finger lands on the center of this high point is where you will find the point.

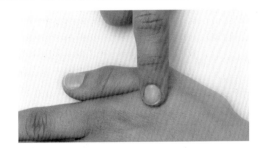

4 Be sure to relax the thumb before pressing the point.

✳ **Warning:** Avoid during pregnancy — can cause contractions.

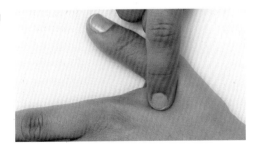

Other Acupressure Points to Consider

After pressing the best acupressure point for this condition, follow with one of these points:

- For apex headache, add **BL-67 / Zhiyin** (see Bladder 67, page 131)
- For temporal headache, add **GB-20 / Fengchi** (see Gallbladder 20, page 140)

Heartburn, Acid Reflux (GERD)

Heartburn, or acid reflux. often referred to as GERD (gastroesophageal reflux disease), is the condition of stomach acid flowing back through the lower esophageal sphincter and into the esophagus and throat, causing burning and irritation.

Most commonly associated with stress, acid reflux can be brought on by foods, medications, anxiety or other triggers. Often the condition will aggravate itself — as the acid rises, the tender tissue of the esophagus will create a thickened area for protection. Individuals with hiatal hernia often experience GERD as a symptom — as the stomach pushes up through the lower esophageal sphincter, it is no longer able to close off the stomach from the esophagus, which results in increased stomach acid outside of the stomach.

SIGNS AND SYMPTOMS

Most commonly, the symptoms are a burning or foul taste in the mouth. There may also be burning and pain in the esophagus, which is often felt in the chest. Usually these symptoms arise fairly quickly after encountering a trigger. There is less desire for food or drink because they will worsen the symptoms. Some people experience an increase in salivation when reflux is triggered.

NOTE

The symptoms listed above often mimic the symptoms of a heart attack (myocardial infarction). Be sure to see a doctor if the symptoms do not change or get worse.

Conception Vessel 12 (CV-12 / Zhongwan)

This point is located on the abdomen.

1 To locate the point, stand in front of a mirror. Expose the abdomen.

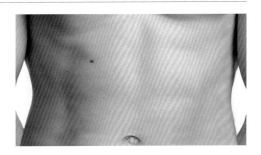

2 Slide the index finger to locate the bottom of the xiphoid process, the lower end of the breastbone (sternum). If the xiphoid itself cannot be located, find the point where the ribs join the low end of the breastbone as a reference point.

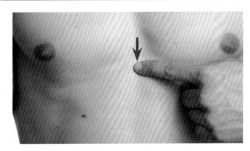

3 Next, locate the belly button (umbilicus).

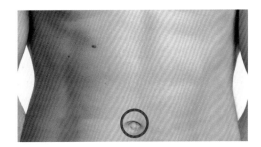

4 The midway point between these two structures, about six fingers' width down from the sternum or up from the belly button, is where you will find the point.

✳ **Warning:** Avoid during pregnancy — may cause too much pressure on the baby.

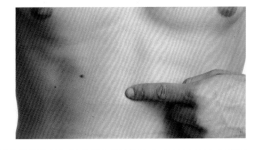

Other Acupressure Points to Consider

After pressing the best acupressure point for this condition, follow with one of these points:

- For heartburn with spasm, add **CV-22 / Tiantu** (see Conception Vessel 22, page 149)
- For heartburn with bloating, add **ST-36 / Zusanli** (see Stomach 36, page 119)

Hiccup

Hiccup is spasm of the diaphragm that causes a characteristic sound.

Eating too much or not eating enough can both lead to hiccups, as can excessive alcohol intake. Smoking may exacerbate a bout of the hiccups. In some people, the condition may arise in stressful situations. The vagus nerve innervates the diaphragm and thus lies at the root of the problem — diseases of the central nervous system may have hiccup as a symptom.

SIGNS AND SYMPTOMS

The condition itself is the main symptom. While the condition is mostly harmless, extended bouts of hiccupping can lead to pain, acid reflux, nausea, vomiting, a cramp in the diaphragm (the muscle involved in breathing that lies below the ribs) and exhaustion.

Eating the first bite of a meal very slowly may help stop the spasm from happening.

OTHER TREATMENTS
- Peppermint oil capsules may help, but see a doctor if the symptoms do not abate.

Lung 10 (LU-10 / Yuji)

This point is located on the palm of the hand, on the thenar eminence (the fleshy base of the thumb).

1 To locate the point, find the thenar eminence on the palm of the hand, the fleshy mound at the base of the thumb.

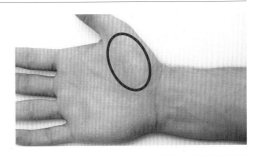

2 Locate the metacarpal bone of the thumb (the bone that connects the thumb to the wrist) that defines the lower edge of the fleshy mound and is found in between the first joint of the thumb and the wrist.

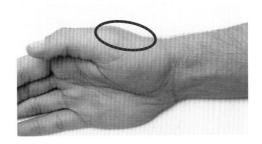

3 Next, slide the tip of the index finger along the metacarpal bone to the midway of the bone, approximately halfway between the wrist and the first joint of the thumb.

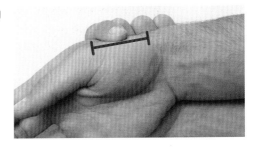

4 The point is located between the bone and the muscles that make up the thenar eminence. Slide the finger over the curve of the bone. Where the finger lands on the space between the bone and the muscles of the mound is where you will find the point.

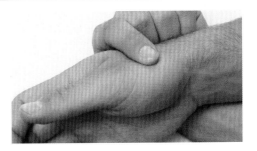

Other Acupressure Points to Consider

After pressing the best acupressure point for this condition, follow with one of these points:

- For hiccup with pain, add **CV-12 / Zhongwan** (see Conception Vessel 12, page 148)

- For hiccup before meals, add **CV-23 / Lianquan** (see Conception Vessel 23, page 150)

Indigestion

Indigestion mostly describes the pain or discomfort that occurs when there is difficulty digesting foods.

Indigestion has nearly as many causes as there are cases; for example, it may occur as a reaction to certain foods, because of a lack of specific digestive enzymes, during a microbial infection, because of bad food or poor food combinations, from injury, surgery, stress and more. In addition, other digestive diseases often exhibit indigestion as a symptom.

SIGNS AND SYMPTOMS

Cramping, stabbing, shooting or dull pain in the abdomen, gas and bloating, diarrhea, nausea, vomiting and acid reflux are common symptoms. Some may also experience irritability or fatigue.

While indigestion seems relatively benign, in some cases it may be a sign of a more serious condition. Alcoholism can lead to indigestion, as can drug abuse, mental health conditions, ulcers, gastric diseases and tumors.

ABDOMINAL MASSAGE
Lie on your left side. Starting at the lower right quadrant (near the top of the right hip bone), slowly and gently massage around the abdomen, in small circular motions, moving up the right side, across under the ribs and down the left side until the discomfort is relieved.

Spleen 4 (SP-4 / Gongsun)

This point is located on the inner side of the foot.

1 To locate the point, sit in a chair and cross one ankle over the opposite knee to allow easy access to the foot. Locate the large protruding bone at the first joint of the big toe.

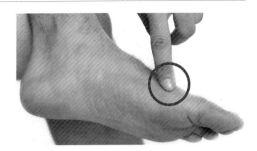

2 With an index finger, roll off the large bone diagonally, in the direction of the bottom of the foot until you feel the first long thin metatarsal bone.

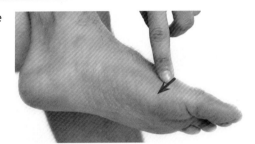

3 Next, slide the finger along the metatarsal bone toward the ankle. You should feel the large tendon on the bottom of the foot on the other side of your finger.

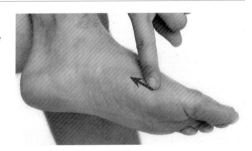

4 Continue to slide the index finger along the first metatarsal bone. Where it lands on a depression between the tendon of the foot and the upper end of the first metatarsal bone is where you will find the point.

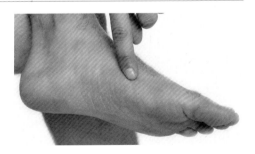

Other Acupressure Points to Consider

After pressing the best acupressure point for this condition, follow with one of these points:

- For indigestion with abdominal pain, add **CV-10 / Xiawan** (see Conception Vessel 10, page 147)

- For indigestion with food stagnation, add **CV-12 / Zhongwan** (see Conception Vessel 12, page 148)

Insomnia

Insomnia is a disrupted sleep cycle and can present as trouble falling asleep or trouble staying asleep.

There are many different reasons why this condition arises, such as stress, anxiety, diet, stimulation, hormonal imbalances, dreams and more.

SIGNS AND SYMPTOMS

Symptoms vary in both presentation and severity from person to person. There may be fatigue or there may be restlessness. Some insomniacs have long stretches of sleeplessness, while others may sleep in short, insufficient blocks of time with short periods of waking in between.

The body's levels of cortisol and melatonin throughout the day form a cycle that determines how we sleep. If either level is out of balance, insomnia will result — and these cycles can be influenced by our behavior choices.

Lack of sleep usually results in irritability and decreased attention or focus. Driving may be impaired if insomnia is extreme. If the condition is chronic, health may generally deteriorate as the body is denied long, uninterrupted sleep, the period of the sleep cycle when the body usually takes care of repair and maintenance.

BREAKING INSOMNIA PATTERNS

Some of the following suggestions can help keep the sleep cycle normal:

- No screen time 1 hour before bed.
- No stimulants, especially caffeine, at least 1 hour before bed.
- Use only soft, warm lighting at night. Try to block all light filtering into the bedroom.
- Set a regular bedtime and stick to it.

Gallbladder 20 (GB-20 / Fengchi)

This point is located on the back of the head.

1 To locate the point, find the bony prominence at the back of the head, about one hand's width above the back hairline.

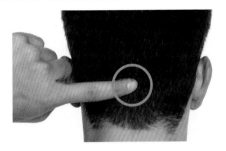

2 Slide the tip of the index finger over this prominence until it lands on a depression.

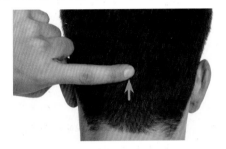

3 Next, move the index finger to the outer side along the bony ridge about three fingers' width, until it hits a fleshy mound.

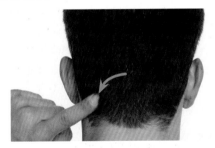

4 Where the finger lands in the center of this mound is where you will find the point.

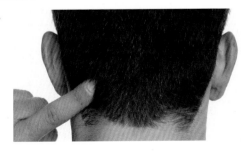

Other Acupressure Points to Consider

After pressing the best acupressure point for this condition, follow with one of these points:

- For insomnia with inability to stop worrying, add **Yintang** (see page 152)

- For insomnia with feeling of not being grounded, add **KI-1 / Yongquan** (see Kidney 1, page 132)

Irregular Menstruation

Irregular menstruation describes a menstrual cycle that is not proceeding on its established normal rhythm.

As every woman may have a different "normal," the definition includes these unique variations. Irregularities are most commonly triggered by hormonal shifts but may be due to changes in nutritional status, increased exercise, injury or stress. Some medications may affect the cycle, while pregnancy will stop the cycle altogether.

SIGNS AND SYMPTOMS

Typical cycles are between 21 and 35 days apart. At the onset of menstruation (menarche), there may be fluctuations in many aspects of the cycle as the body adjusts to the changes in hormonal levels. Another time of natural change is perimenopause, the time around the onset of menopause. (Menopause is defined as 365 days since the last period. On the 366th day, the status is defined as post-menopause).

The irregularity of the rhythm may be associated with the length of time between cycles of bleeding or the number of days on which bleeding occurs. It may indicate a change in flow, either more or less volume, or breakout bleeding between cycles. Finally, it may manifest as a change of symptoms, such as increased pain or mood swings.

NOTE

A sudden or dramatic change could indicate a more serious condition and should be diagnosed as soon as possible.

Spleen 10 (SP-10 / Xuehai)

This point is located on the inner leg just above the knee.

1 To locate the point, extend your legs while seated on a bed or floor.

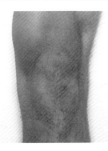

2 Place the index and middle fingers of one hand horizontally across the leg above the knee, so that the lower edge of the middle finger sits on the upper margin of the kneecap. The second joint of both fingers should be right above the center of the kneecap.

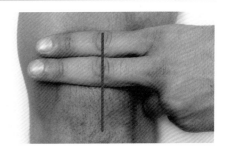

3 Next, slide the index finger toward the inner thigh about 1 inch (2.5 cm), so that the tip of the index finger lands about 1 inch further down the curve of the inner thigh than it was.

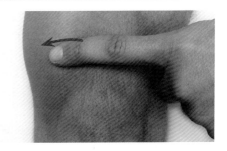

4 Where the tip of the index finger lands on a slight depression is where you will find the point.

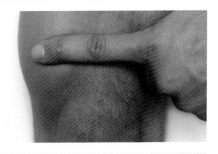

Other Acupressure Points to Consider

After pressing the best acupressure point for this condition, follow with one of these points:

- Also add **LR-3 / Taichong** (see Liver 3, page 144)
- For irregular menstruation with cramping and pain, add **SP-8 / Diji** (see Spleen 8, page 123)

Menopausal Symptoms

Hot flashes — the sensation of heat, commonly moving in a wave over the body — is the symptom most associated with the hormonal changes of menopause.

Stress, spicy food, caffeine, smoking and alcohol have all been shown to worsen hot flashes. Women who exercise regularly tend to experience hot flashes less often and less severely than sedentary women.

SIGNS AND SYMPTOMS

In addition to the heat, there may be dizziness and a prickling sensation on the skin. Sweating is common, especially at night; in severe cases, the sheets may have to be changed several times in one night.

Post-menopausal women often experience another symptom — vaginal dryness. In fact, dryness can manifest in many ways, including skin, hair and eyes. Some women report a decreased interest in sexual activity, due in part to the discomfort from dryness. Urinary incontinence is common, and may be accompanied by increased urgency and frequency.

OTHER TREATMENTS
- A topical cream made from wild yam (Dioscorea villosa) may help with vaginal dryness.
- Increasing the fat-soluble vitamins (A, E, and especially D) can be helpful for reducing menopausal symptoms as well.
- Consider adding more calcium-rich foods like kale, tofu, or sardines to the diet.

Kidney 6 (KI-6 / Zhaohai)

This point is located on the inner foot below the inner ankle bone.

1 To locate the point, sit in a chair and cross one ankle over the opposite knee to allow easy access to the ankle.

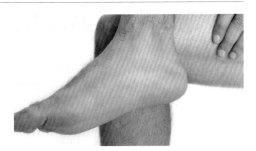

2 Locate your inner ankle bone.

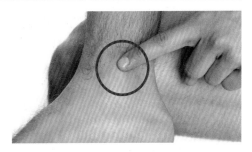

3 Next, from there, slide the tip of the index finger from the ankle bone down, until it drops into a depression located about one thumb's width below the bone.

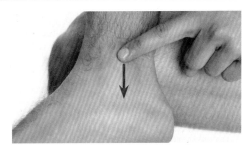

4 Where the finger lands on this depression is where you will find the point.

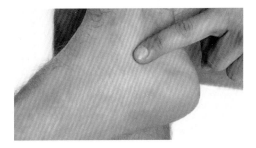

Other Acupressure Points to Consider

After pressing the best acupressure point for this condition, follow with one of these points:

- Also add **SP-6 / Sanyinjiao** (see Spleen 6, page 122)

- For menopausal symptoms with urinary incontinence, add **CV-4 / Guanyuan** (see Conception Vessel 4, page 146)

Morning Sickness

Morning sickness is an increase in nausea during pregnancy.

It is caused by the radical shift in hormones that characterize pregnancy.

A variant of this condition is referred to as hyperemesis gravidarum, which is a much more serious condition. It involves constant and unrelenting nausea and the inability to keep anything, often even water, in the system. It can lead to dehydration and electrolyte imbalances — very alarming symptoms any time, but especially when pregnant. Moms experiencing hyperemesis gravidarum often require hospitalization and intravenous nutrients and fluids.

SIGNS AND SYMPTOMS

The nausea is usually accompanied by vomiting, which often relieves the nausea. There may be accompanying symptoms of headache, dizziness, fatigue or sweating.

NOTE

The protocols outlined here may help prevent or lessen morning sickness but are not appropriate for the much more serious hyperemesis gravidarum.

Pericardium 6 (PC-6 / Neiguan)

This point is located on the inner forearm close to the wrist.

1 To locate the point, rest the arm on a comfortable surface, palm side facing up.

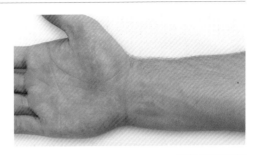

2 Place two middle fingers from your left hand on your right forearm so that the middle finger lays facedown over the wrist crease. Where the index finger falls is the horizontal location line. Note the line and remove your left hand from your forearm.

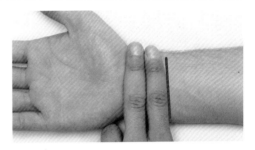

3 Next, locate the tendon in the center of the forearm by bending your hand at the wrist so that the palm is moving up, toward the elbow.

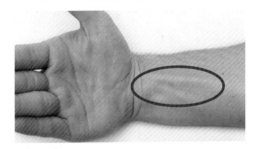

4 Where the horizontal location line intersects the tendon is where you will find the point. Bring your hand back down before pressing the point.

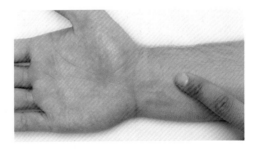

Other Acupressure Points to Consider

After pressing the best acupressure point for this condition, follow with one of these points:

- For morning sickness with headache, add **ST-8 / Touwei** (see Stomach 8, page 117)

- For morning sickness with weakness, add **SP-6 / Sanyinjiao** (see Spleen 6, page 122)

Nausea and Vomiting

Nausea is a sensation often resulting in a need to vomit. Vomiting is the body's technique for removing matter from the upper gastrointestinal tract very quickly

Both nausea and vomiting may result from ingesting bad food or allergens, overeating or overindulging in alcohol. Due to motion sickness, some people experience both when traveling.

SIGNS AND SYMPTOMS

Nausea leads to a queasy, unsettled feeling in the abdomen. There may be sweating, shaking, dizziness or fatigue. Increased salivation and activation of the gag reflex often precede the act of vomiting. Vomiting can result in sore throat, irritation and burning as stomach acid comes into prolonged contact with the tissues of the throat and mouth.

Rapid onset violent vomiting is a common sign of food poisoning. It may also signal trauma to the head, heart or digestive system. It may indicate internal bleeding, especially if there is blood in the vomit.

NOTE

If vomiting is excessive or ongoing, it commonly leads to dehydration requiring hospitalization for IV fluids.

SLOW-BREATHING TIP

Always take three deep, slow, relaxing breaths before eating. This activates the parasympathetic state (also called "rest and digest").

Pericardium 6 (PC-6 / Neiguan)

This point is located on the inner forearm close to the wrist.

1 To locate the point, rest the arm on a comfortable surface, palm side facing up.

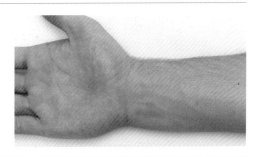

2 Place two middle fingers from your left hand on your right forearm so that the middle finger lays facedown over the wrist crease. Where the index finger falls is the horizontal location line. Note the line and remove your left hand from your forearm.

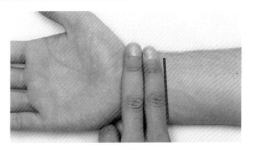

3 Next, locate the tendon in the center of the forearm by bending your hand at the wrist so that the palm is moving up, toward the elbow.

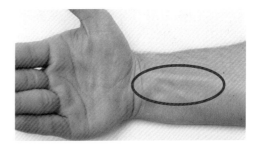

4 Where the horizontal location line intersects the tendon is where you will find the point. Bring your hand back down before pressing the point.

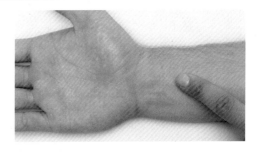

Other Acupressure Points to Consider

After pressing the best acupressure point for this condition, follow with one of these points:

- For nausea and vomiting with food stagnation, add **CV-12 / Zhongwan** (see Conception Vessel 12, page 148)

- For nausea and vomiting with burping and indigestion, add **SP-4 / Gongsun** (see Spleen 4, page 121)

Neck Spasm, Stiff Neck (Torticollis)

Stiff neck is an extremely common condition most people have felt at some point in their lives.

It is often a result of overuse or poor posture. Sleeping positions often lead to a stiff neck upon awakening.

Torticollis is a more severe condition of stiff neck associated with muscle spasm or contraction, and is usually chronic. Torticollis may be genetic or could be due to a traumatic injury.

SIGNS AND SYMPTOMS

Stiff neck symptoms include muscle tension, stiffness and usually pain. It may be accompanied by headache, eye pain or shoulder pain.

Torticollis looks like an exaggerated version of the same symptoms. There is often torsion (twisting) and a dramatically reduced range of motion. In some cases, there may be tonic torticollis, which is little to no motion as the contracted muscle locks up the whole neck. On the other hand, there may be involuntary movements like shaking or twitching, known as clonic torticollis. The pain may be extreme.

NOTE

Torticollis may require medical intervention to relax the contracted muscle. The condition is often treated with Botox injections, which "paralyze" the muscle so that it cannot contract.

STRETCHING THE NECK

It is imperative that the muscles of the neck be gently stretched on a daily basis. A physical therapist can help with exercises specifically for torticollis.

Small Intestine 3 (SI-3 / Houxi)

This point is located on the outer side of the hand.

1 To locate the point, slide the tip of the index finger along the pinky finger toward the wrist.

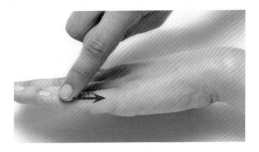

2 Slide the tip of the finger over the first joint of the pinky finger and onto a depression on the outer side of the hand.

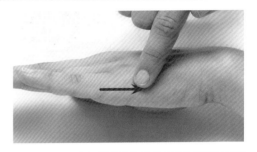

3 The depression lies between the pad on the outer edge of the palm (the hypothenar eminence) and the long bone along the side of the hand (the metacarpal of the pinky finger).

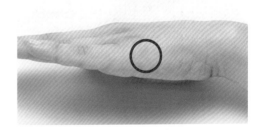

4 Where the finger lands on the center of this depression is where you will find the point.

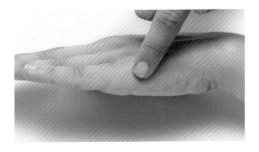

Other Acupressure Points to Consider

After pressing the best acupressure point for this condition, follow with one of these points:

- Also add **LU-7 / Lieque** (see Lung 7, page 108)

- For torticollis with stiff neck, add **GB-20 / Fengchi** (see Gallbladder 20, page 140) if the pain is in the scalenes on the side of the neck

Phlegm

Phlegm is another name for mucus, the substance that lines the mucous membranes of the body, especially those of the gastrointestinal and respiratory systems.

The function of mucus is to moisturize and lubricate the tissues where it is found; this is usually the work of thinner mucus secretions. Mucus contains its own immune factors, substances such as antibodies and enzymes, that recognize pathogens and tag them for removal or break them down at the site.

SIGNS AND SYMPTOMS

The main sign is excess, thickened mucus in the respiratory system, with an increased tendency to cough. Phlegm is most commonly seen in the digestive system when an enema or colonic is used, as the water removes stuck phlegm from the colon.

In the respiratory tract, mucus usually leads to coughing up more phlegm as the lung work to expel the mucus. In the digestive tract, mucus that dries out and thickens can lead to increased symptoms of constipation.

If the phlegm is very stubborn, the body's attempts to expel it may cause injuries. Coughing, for example, may lead to a sore throat or, in extreme cases, prolapse of organs such as the bladder or uterus as the increase in pressure bears down and weakens the connective tissues.

Stomach 40 (ST-40 / Fenglong)

This point is located on the lower leg.

1 To locate the point, sit in a chair with both feet flat on the ground and the knees bent. Find the lower edge of the kneecap (patella). This is the upper location line. Note the line.

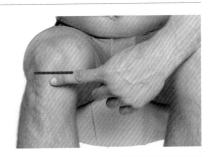

2 Next, locate the front ankle crease. To find this line, with the index finger held horizontally, slide it from the toes up the foot until it runs into the ankle, right before the 90-degree bend created by the lower leg. This is the lower location line.

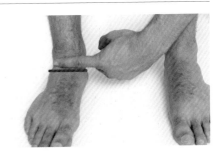

3 Next, slide the index finger down from the upper location line, along the shinbone (tibia) to find the midpoint between these two lines — it should be around two-hands width down from the upper location line.

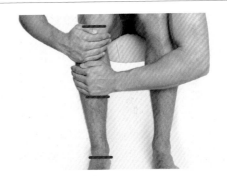

4 Slide the index finger to the outer side of the lower leg along a horizontal line two fingers' width. This is where you will find the point.

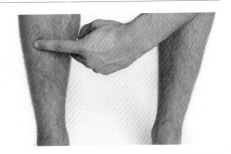

Other Acupressure Points to Consider

After pressing the best acupressure point for this condition, follow with one of these points:

- For excessive respiratory phlegm production, add **LU-11 / Shaoshang** (see Lung 11, page 110)
- For respiratory phlegm with lack of energy to cough, add **LU-7 / Lieque** (see Lung 7, page 108)

Pinkeye (Conjunctivitis)

Conjunctivitis is an inflammation of the conjunctiva of the eye.

This condition is often referred to by its common name, pinkeye, and may be caused by bacterial or viral agents, or by irritation from pollutants or allergens. Contact lens wearers often develop pinkeye from the lens itself, especially if the lenses are old or degraded.

SIGNS AND SYMPTOMS

Reddening of the conjunctiva, excessive tearing, itching, burning eyes and blurred vision are possible symptoms of the condition. If pinkeye is due to an infectious agent, there may be a yellow or green discharge.

If the condition is caused by an infectious agent, antibiotics are usually prescribed. Because many of the bacteria that cause conjunctivitis can be quite damaging, it is important to see a doctor.

NOTE

As pinkeye is primarily caused by bacteria, it is important to wash hands well before and after pressing. It can be more effective to treat the uninfected eye, but if both are infected wear disposable gloves when pressing.

Bladder 1 (BL-1 / Jingming)

This point is located on the face, in between the nose and the inner corner of the eye (inner canthus), and slightly above it.

① To locate the point, look at your face in a mirror.

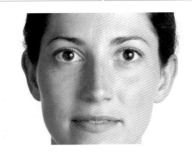

② Locate the inner canthus, the area where the two eyelids come together, close to the nose.

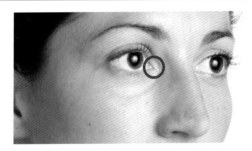

③ Next, gently place an index finger over the inner eyelid until the tip of the finger is resting in the inner canthus.

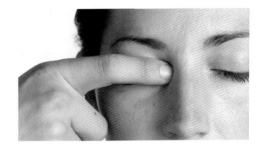

④ Very gently apply pressure to the eyeball while rolling the tip of the finger over it until the fingertip rolls over the innermost edge of the bone of the eye socket. Where the finger falls into the gap between the eyeball and the bone of the eye socket is where you will find the point. This point is held, not pressed.

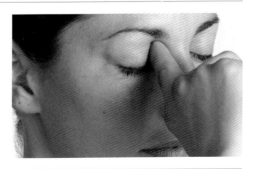

Other Acupressure Points to Consider

After pressing the best acupressure point for this condition, follow with one of these points:

- For conjunctivitis with eye pain, add
  BL-2 / Zanzhu (see Bladder 2, page 129)

Runny or Stuffy Nose (Rhinitis)

A stuffy nose and a runny nose both result from inflammation of the nasal passages.

A stuffy or runny nose is a common sign of many different conditions, including a cold, flu, allergies and sinus infection, which all commonly lead to drainage symptoms. Inhaling an irritant will stimulate this natural defense, which works to remove the irritant.

SIGNS AND SYMPTOMS

With a stuffy nose, the inflammation is so great it is restricting the flow of mucus, whereas with a runny nose, the increased secretions are more obvious. Typically, secretions are clear, watery and copious. Tearing of the eyes is a common accompanying symptom. If a runny nose continues long enough, it can lead to irritation of the tissues, both in the nose and below it, as well as on the nostrils.

If the mucus changes in color or becomes dark, it is usually a sign of infection. Bleeding may be a sign of irritated tissue or a more serious problem.

NASAL WASH

Cleansing the sinuses with a neti pot, nasal syringe or nasal spray may help. To prepare the formula to treat thin clear secretions, add 1/2 teaspoon (2 mL) of apple cider vinegar to 1/2 cup (125 mL) of warm water and add it to the device. For thick secretions, add 1/4 teaspoon (1 mL) of salt to 1/2 cup (125 mL) of warm water and add to the device. Follow the directions for the device used.

Large Intestine 20 (LI-20 / Yingxiang)

This point is located on the face, very close to the nose.

1 To locate the point, look at your face in a mirror.

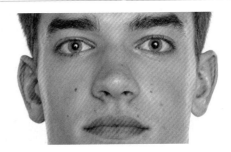

2 Place the tip of the index finger in the nasolabial groove, the area between the outer edge of the nostril and the upper lip.

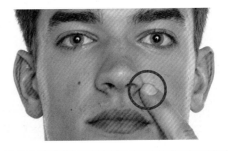

3 It may help to smile when locating the groove.

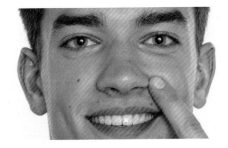

4 Where the finger falls at the top of the groove, closest to the nostril, is where you will find the point.

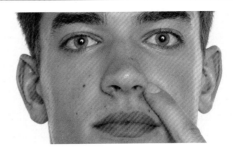

Other Acupressure Points to Consider

After pressing the best acupressure point for this condition, follow with one of these points:

- For rhinitis with tearing eyes, add **BL-2 / Zanzhu** (see Bladder 2, page 129)

- For rhinitis with constant draining, add **GV-20 / Baihui** (see Governing Vessel 20, page 151)

Sciatica

As a condition, sciatica describes pain that originates deep in the posterior pelvic girdle and radiates along the sciatic nerve, which runs down the back of the leg.

The pain of sciatica is due to an odd anomaly of anatomy — the sciatic nerve runs between two muscles, the piriformis and obturator. If either muscle becomes inflamed, the nerve is trapped, leading to pain from the pressure. Sciatica usually occurs on one side of the body but can happen in both legs at the same time.

SIGNS AND SYMPTOMS

The primary symptom is pain, especially down the back of either leg. Other symptoms include tingling and numbness, which often occurs in the "saddle" region — the buttocks and inner thighs. Shooting electric sensations, lessened reflexes and reduced function of the affected side are common.

If sciatica occurs in both legs at the same time or results in incontinence, it can be a condition called cauda equina syndrome. This is a much more serious condition of inflammation of the nerve roots deep in the spine — see a doctor.

Gallbladder 30 (GB-30 / Huantiao)

This point is located on the buttocks.

1 To locate the point, stand in a relaxed position.

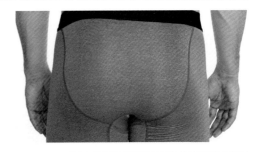

2 With your fingers, find the large depression at the center of one of the buttock cheeks.

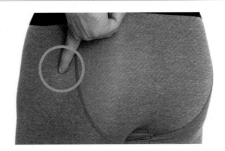

3 This point falls on a line drawn from the tip of the tailbone (coccyx) to the hip socket.

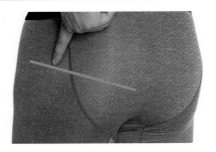

4 Where the finger lands on the center of this depression is where you will find the point.

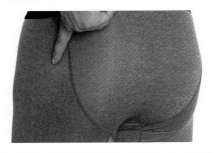

Other Acupressure Points to Consider

After pressing the best acupressure point for this condition, follow with one of these points:

- For sciatica with numbness, add **KI-3 / Taixi** (see Kidney 3, page 133)

- For sciatica with low back pain, add **BL-40 / Weizhong** (see Bladder 40, page 130)

Skin Blemishes (Acne)

If a skin blemish is simply a clogged pore, it is called a blackhead or whitehead. If the irritation becomes infected and inflamed, usually as a result of bacterial infection, it is a pimple. Acne is a combination of all of these, and may also involve painful cysts under the skin.

Skin irritations occur when the skin is not efficiently turning over skin cells or processing sebum, resulting in clogged pores. Acne may arise because of hormonal changes, stress, changes in diet or other reasons. Skin eruptions can result from changes in beneficial bacteria that exist naturally on the skin. Ironically, overly harsh cleansing products designed specifically to eradicate blemishes may cause these changes.

Some medications may kill off the healthy, protective bacteria that lives on our skin. Irritations, such as scrubbing the skin too vigorously or tight clothing rubbing on the skin, can also lead to eruptions. Dietary choices may increase the likelihood of developing skin problems and dietary changes may help reverse the situation. Allergies are also frequently seen to cause skin imbalances. Certain nutritional deficiencies, especially of fat-soluble vitamins such as vitamin A and E, are also known to cause blemishes.

SIGNS AND SYMPTOMS

Skin blemishes can appear anywhere on the body, especially where nutritional deficiencies are involved. Vitamin A deficiency rash commonly appears on the back of the upper arms, and vitamin B deficiency is the cause of pellagra.

Irritated skin should always be handled gently. What is needed in most cases is simply cleaning and treating the skin oils to achieve clearer skin. Too much pressure when attempting to extract a blackhead or pimple can lead to permanent damage of the tissue and increase the likelihood of developing acne.

Stomach 7 (ST-7 / Xiaguan)

This point is located on the jaw.

1 To locate the point, look at your face in a mirror.

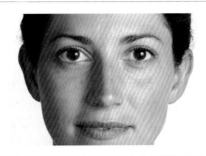

2 Locate the top of the cheekbone and slide an index finger along the outer edge of it toward the ear until it runs into the joint of the jaw. To test that the finger is at the joint, open the mouth wide — it should feel as though the jawbone is pushing the finger out of the depression.

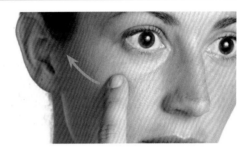

3 The fingertip should be in a depression about one thumb's width from the tragus, the small flap of cartilage at the front of the ear.

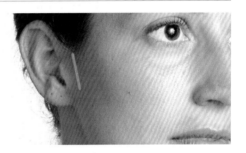

4 The direct center of this depression is where you will find the point.

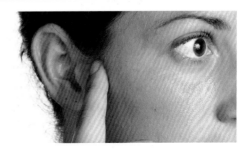

Other Acupressure Points to Consider

After pressing the best acupressure point for this condition, follow with one of these points:

- For skin blemishes with excessive oil production, add **Yintang** (page 152) and **ST-8 / Touwei** (see Stomach 8, page 117)

- For skin blemishes with inflammation, especially on nose, add **LI-20 / Yingxiang** (see Large Intestine 20, page 114)

Sore Throat

Sore throat is most often described as a raw or irritated throat.

The symptoms can appear in different locations; for example, the pharynx (pharyngitis) or larynx (laryngitis). The most common cause of sore throat is viral infection. In fact, sore throat is often the first symptom of a cold or flu.

Sore throat may also result from overuse; singers and public speakers often experience it. Inhalants and pollution can lead to throat irritation, as can post-nasal drip from a cold, allergies or sinus infection. Acid reflux at night may lead to sore throat upon rising.

SIGNS AND SYMPTOMS

Soreness, a raw feeling, burning, swelling and redness are all typical signs of a sore throat. The throat may itch or ache before the other symptoms appear. There may be hoarseness or total loss of voice (laryngitis). Rapid onset, swollen lymph nodes, a fever and a characteristic throat rash are usually reliable indicators to determine whether the sore throat is from a strep infection.

NOTE

Some people develop an ache in the throat when fatigued. This may be linked to thyroid dysfunction and should be checked out. If strep throat is suspected or if the sore throat is accompanied by a fever over 102°F (38.9°C), see a doctor for a diagnosis.

Kidney 6 (KI-6 / Zhaohai)

This point is located on the inner foot below the inner ankle bone.

1 To locate the point, sit in a chair and cross one ankle over the opposite knee to allow easy access to the ankle.

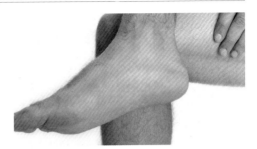

2 Locate your inner ankle bone.

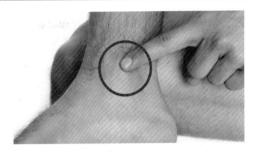

3 Next, from there, slide the tip of the index finger from the ankle bone down, until it drops into a depression located about one thumb's width below the bone.

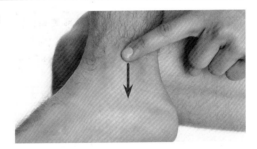

4 Where the finger lands on this depression is where you will find the point.

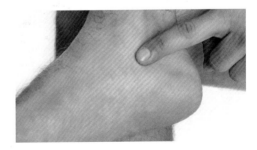

Other Acupressure Points to Consider

After pressing the best acupressure point for this condition, follow with one of these points:

- For sore throat due to virus, add **LU-11 / Shaoshang** (see Lung 11, page 110)

- For sore throat with laryngitis, add **CV-23 / Lianquan** (see Conception Vessel 23, page 150)

Tennis Elbow, Golfer's Elbow (Epicondylitis)

Epicondylitis is the name given to pain that occurs in the elbow.

It usually occurs from overuse, or repetitive actions; swinging a racquet or club is a common cause, as the name suggests. It is often seen in those not playing either sport — mechanics, factory workers, professional cleaners and weavers regularly develop epicondylitis.

With this condition, repetition further irritates already inflamed tissues. Tennis elbow happens when the outer side is painful, and golfer's elbow occurs on the inner side.

SIGNS AND SYMPTOMS

Pain is the primary — and in many cases only — symptom. The pain is usually a constant ache, exacerbated by the same motions that led to the condition. The pain is worse with gripping, lifting or twisting; for example, opening a jar may be painful. Stiffness and a significant decrease in range of motion are common.

It is crucial to stop the activity that led to the problem so that tissues can heal, although this can be difficult if the activities are part of daily living or one's work.

Large Intestine 11 (LI-11 / Quchi)

This point is located on the forearm, very close to the elbow.

1 To locate the point, bend the arm 90 degrees.

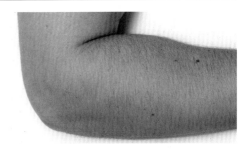

2 With the tip of the index finger from the opposite hand, locate the outermost end of the elbow crease.

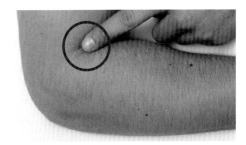

3 Next, slide the finger (away from the body) three fingers' width toward the elbow bone to locate the bony prominence (olecranon process) of the elbow, closest to the elbow crease.

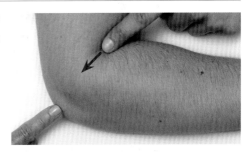

4 Where the finger lands on the midpoint between the elbow crease and the olecranon process is where you will find the point.

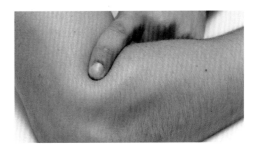

Other Acupressure Points to Consider

After pressing the best acupressure point for this condition, follow with one of these points:

- For epicondylitis radiating down the arm, add **TW-3 / Zhongzhu** (see Triple Warmer 3, page 138)
- For epicondylitis radiating up the arm, add **TW-14 / Jianliao** (see Triple Warmer 14, page 139)

Toothache

Toothache may be a symptom of tooth decay, in particular when the decay reaches the nerve of the tooth and sends a pain signal.

A cracked tooth will also lead to pain. Poor circulation to the gums may lead to weak, sensitive teeth. Temporomandibular joint (TMJ) syndrome, a misalignment of the jaw due to injury or repetitive motion, often results in pain that may be difficult to distinguish from tooth decay. It is a good idea to get a diagnosis from a doctor or dentist because the conditions are treated quite differently.

SIGNS AND SYMPTOMS

Pain is the main symptom. It may be difficult or impossible to chew with the teeth on the painful side. If the source of the problem is infection, there may be swelling and redness. It is possible to see infected discharge around the decaying tooth, usually accompanied by a foul odor.

CAUTION: Clove oil can be used sparingly to temporarily reduce tooth pain. Do not use more than three drops a day for no more than a few days at most.

Kidney 3 (KI-3 / Taixi)

This point is located on the inner ankle.

1 To locate the point, sit in a chair and cross one ankle over the opposite knee to allow easy access to the ankle.

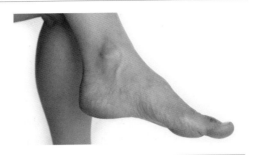

2 Locate the highest point of the inner ankle bone.

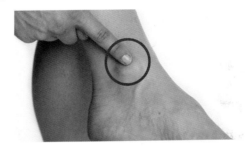

3 Next, from there, slide the tip of the index finger back toward the Achilles tendon, the large tendon that connects the calf to the foot, until the finger lands on a depression.

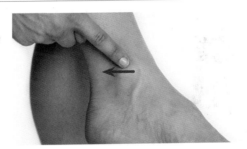

4 Where the finger lands on the center of this depression is where you will find the point.

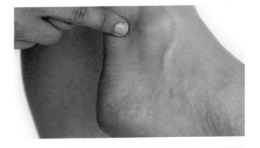

Other Acupressure Points to Consider

After pressing the best acupressure point for this condition, follow with one of these points:

- For toothache in the top teeth, add **ST-7 / Xiaguan** (see Stomach 7, page 116)

- For toothache in the bottom teeth, add **ST-6 / Jiache** (Stomach 6, see page 115) with **LU-10 / Yuji** (see Lung 10, page 109)

Urinary Incontinence

Urinary incontinence is an increasing difficulty with keeping urine in the bladder.

The condition has many causes: age, surgery, nerve damage, lack of tone (not enough exercise), obesity, pregnancy and childbirth, stress and urinary tract infections. As the bladder is controlled by parasympathetic branches of the lower spinal nerves, an injury to the back could result in incontinence. Cystitis, bladder and kidney infections all have incontinence as a symptom.

SIGNS AND SYMPTOMS

Incontinence that occurs with age or injury is usually painless, but if there is an infection, burning and pain upon urination is common. Incontinence often begins with small leaks when laughing, coughing or sneezing, and it becomes more difficult to stop the flow in midstream. Bedwetting, or nocturnal enuresis, is the inability to control the bladder at night.

NOTE

If incontinence comes on suddenly or is accompanied by persistent numbness or tingling, it could be a sign of a more serious condition and should be diagnosed by a doctor.

OTHER TREATMENTS
- Exercises that strengthen the pelvic floor, such as Kegel exercises, may help
- Avoid triggers, such as alcohol, caffeine, sugar and spicy foods, that may worsen the situation

Conception Vessel 4 (CV-4 / Guanyuan)

This point is located on the lower abdomen.

1 To locate the point, stand in front of a mirror. Expose the lower abdomen.

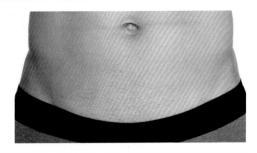

2 Locate the belly button (umbilicus). Place a finger on it.

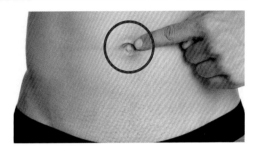

3 Next, slide the finger down about four fingers' width.

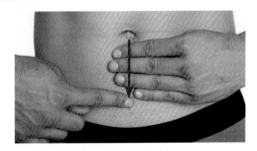

4 Where the finger lands on the swell of tissue just under the belly button is where you will find the point.

✳ **Warning:** Avoid during pregnancy — may cause too much pressure on the baby.

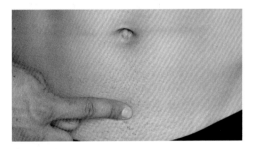

Other Acupressure Points to Consider

After pressing the best acupressure point for this condition, follow with one of these points:

- For urinary incontinence due to prolapse, add **SP-6 / Sanyinjiao** (see Spleen 6, page 122)

- For urinary incontinence with burning, add **LR-3 / Taichong** (see Liver 3, page 144)

Vaginal Discharge (Leukorrhea)

Leukorrhea is another name for vaginal discharge.

It is usually white, although it may appear yellowish. The discharge is mostly mucus and may contain pus or blood. It may occur regularly or appear suddenly. Hormonal imbalance is commonly the cause, but it may be an indication of another condition, such as a bacterial or fungal vaginal infection.

Sexual intercourse with a new partner may lead to infection as the vaginal flora adjust to the bacterial profile of the new partner. So-called honeymooner's disease is usually cystitis (urinary tract infection) but may manifest as a vaginal infection as well.

SIGNS AND SYMPTOMS

The term "leukorrhea" describes a primary symptom — vaginal discharge. It may be thin to thick, copious or scant, white to yellow. Red-tinged or green discharge is a sign of a more serious condition, especially if the color darkens or it is accompanied by a foul odor. Itching, pain, redness and swelling are common symptoms of a vaginal infection. Although primarily associated with sexually transmitted diseases, odor may occur with all vaginal infections.

> **NOTE**
>
> Leukorrhea may be a sign of an underlying infection. All infections should be speedily addressed, but because many sexually transmitted diseases have serious consequences, they should be treated as soon as possible.

Liver 8 (LR-8 / Ququan)

This point is located on the leg, close to the inner knee.

1 To locate the point, extend the leg and find the bottom edge of the kneecap (patella).

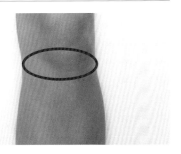

2 Lay four fingers across the kneecap on the opposite leg so that the outer edge of the pinky finger sits at the bottom of the kneecap. The index finger should be resting on a line that extends through the fleshy tissue on the inner leg.

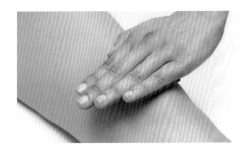

3 Next, slide the tip of the index finger about an inch down the curve of the inner thigh until it is on the highest point of this fleshy area.

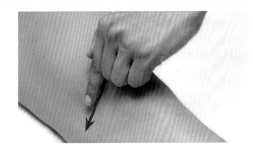

4 Where the tip of the finger rests on this highest point is where you will find the point.

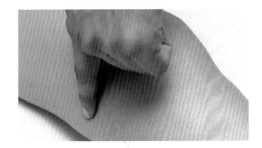

Other Acupressure Points to Consider

After pressing the best acupressure point for this condition, follow with one of these points:

- For vaginal infections and leukorrhea due to yeast, add **SP-8 / Diji** (see Spleen 8, page 123)
- For vaginal infections and leukorrhea with vaginal prolapse, add **SP-10 / Xuehai** (see Spleen 10, page 124)

CHAPTER 3

Acupressure Points

Lung 7 (LU-7 / Lieque)

This point is located on the crest of the forearm, very close to the wrist.

1 To locate the point, rest the hand on a comfortable surface, palm side facing up. Locate the wrist crease by slightly bending the hand up. Relax the hand.

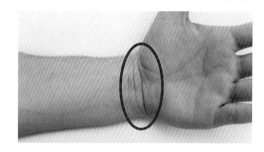

2 With your other hand, lay the three middle fingers horizontally along the crease, with the fourth (ring) finger positioned on the crease itself.

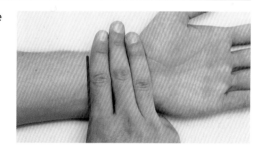

3 Next, roll the tip of the index finger up and over the radius bone, the bone on the thumb side of the forearm.

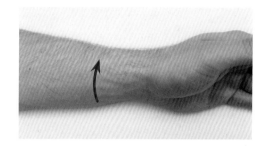

4 Where the tip of the finger lands on the radius bone is where you will find the point.

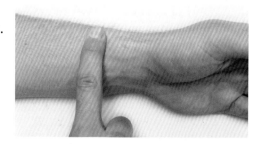

Helps with these conditions

- common cold
- sneezing
- runny nose
- sore throat
- stiff neck

- headache
- frozen shoulder (adhesive capsulitis)
- asthma
- bronchitis

Lung 10 (LU-10 / Yuji)

This point is located on the palm of the hand, on the thenar eminence (the fleshy base of the thumb).

1 To locate the point, find the thenar eminence on the palm of the hand, the fleshy mound at the base of the thumb.

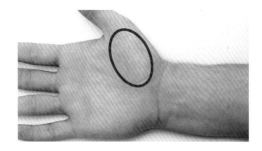

2 Locate the metacarpal bone of the thumb (the bone that connects the thumb to the wrist) that defines the lower edge of the fleshy mound and is found in between the first joint of the thumb and the wrist.

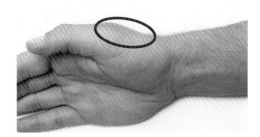

3 Next, slide the tip of the index finger along the metacarpal bone to the midway of the bone, approximately halfway between the wrist and the first joint of the thumb.

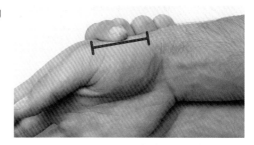

4 The point is located between the bone and the muscles that make up the thenar eminence. Slide the finger over the curve of the bone. Where the finger lands on the space between the bone and the muscles of the mound is where you will find the point.

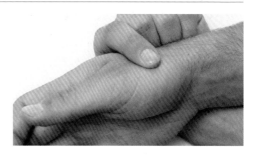

Helps with these conditions

- hiccups
- shortness of breath
- painful cough
- heat and dryness in the chest, nose, throat or lungs
- sore throat
- dry throat

Lung 11 (LU-11 / Shaoshang)

This point is located on the thumb, near the nail.

1 To locate the point, rest the hand on a comfortable surface, palm side facing up, ensuring thumb is elevated.

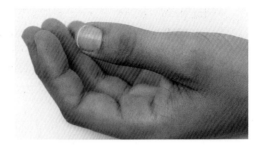

2 Note the line along the bottom of the thumbnail.

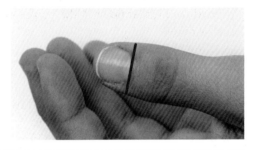

3 Note another line along the outer edge of the nail, the edge farthest from the index finger.

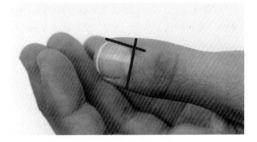

4 Where these two location lines intersect is where you will find the point.

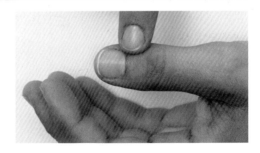

Helps with these conditions

- tennis elbow, golfer's elbow (epicondylitis)
- sore throat
- dry throat
- nosebleeds
- fever in children, especially with childhood diseases

Large Intestine 4 (LI-4 / Hegu)

This point is located on the back side of the hand, near the base of the thumb.

1 To locate the point, move the thumb toward the index finger until the two are pressed together. This will cause a fleshy mound of skin to bunch up on the back of the hand, between the index finger and thumb.

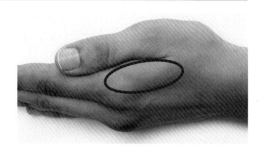

2 Find the highest point at the center of this mound.

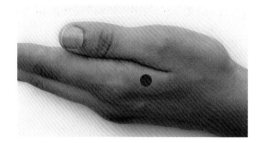

3 Where the finger lands on the center of this high point is where you will find the point.

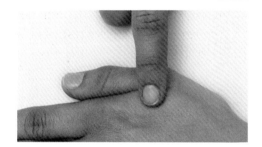

4 Be sure to relax the thumb before pressing the point.

✳ Warning: Avoid during pregnancy — can cause contractions.

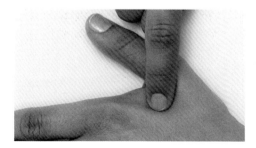

Helps with these conditions

- the first signs of a cold or flu
- headache
- red or hot eyes
- nosebleed
- toothache
- mouth sores
- sore throat
- tinnitus
- bacterial infections
- may speed delivery in childbirth

Large Intestine 11 (LI-11 / Quchi)

This point is located on the forearm, very close to the elbow.

1 To locate the point, bend the arm 90 degrees.

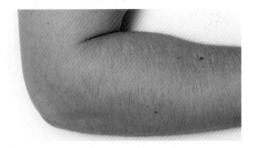

2 With the tip of the index finger from the opposite hand, locate the outermost end of the elbow crease.

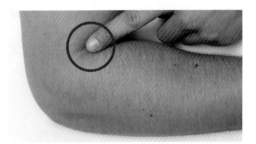

3 Next, slide the finger (away from the body) three fingers' width toward the elbow bone to locate the bony prominence (olecranon process) of the elbow, closest to the elbow crease.

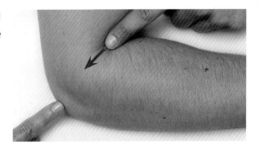

4 Where the finger lands on the midpoint between the elbow crease and the olecranon process is where you will find the point.

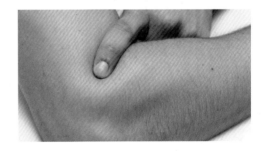

Helps with these conditions

- eczema (atopic dermatitis)
- acne
- any condition of the skin
- fever
- viral infections

Large Intestine 15 (LI-15 / Jianyu)

This point is located on the front of the shoulder.

1. To locate the point, stand in front of a mirror. Bend the arm 90 degrees and raise the elbow until it is level with the shoulder.

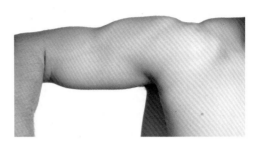

2. This will cause two depressions to appear next to each other at the top of the shoulder. If they are not obvious, palpate for them just above the deltoid muscle at the top of the arm.

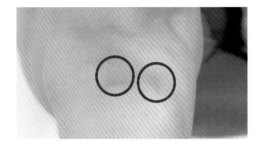

3. Next, use the index finger from the opposite hand to find the depression that is in the front.

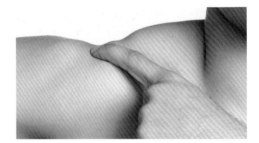

4. Where the finger lands on the depression closest to the chest is where you will find the point. Be sure to relax the arm before pressing the point.

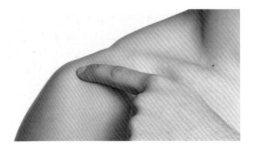

Helps with these conditions

- frozen shoulder (adhesive capsulitis), especially at the front of the shoulder
- any imbalance of the shoulder

Large Intestine 20 (LI-20 / Yingxiang)

This point is located on the face, very close to the nose.

1 To locate the point, look at your face in a mirror.

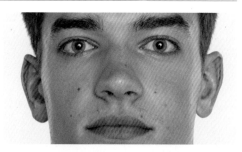

2 Place the tip of the index finger in the nasolabial groove, the area between the outer edge of the nostril and the upper lip.

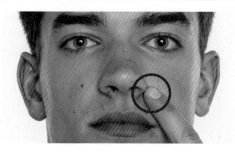

3 It may help to smile when locating the groove.

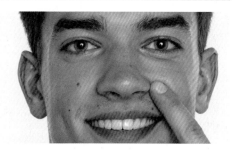

4 Where the finger falls at the top of the groove, closest to the nostril, is where you will find the point.

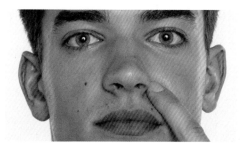

Helps with these conditions

- any condition of the nose
- nasal congestion
- nosebleed
- runny or stuffy nose (rhinitis)
- sneezing
- loss of sense of smell (anosmia)

Stomach 6 (ST-6 / Jiache)

This point is located on the lower jaw.

1 To locate the point, look at your face in a mirror.

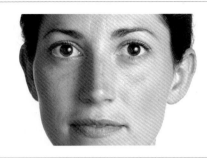

2 Gently clench the teeth and slide an index finger along the lower jawbone from the chin toward the back of the jaw until it finds the mound slightly above the jawbone.

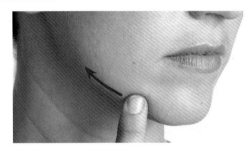

3 To ensure the correct location of the mound, relax the jaw and the mound will disappear.

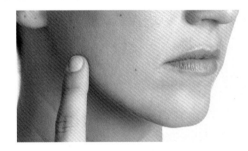

4 The direct center of this mound is where you will find the point.

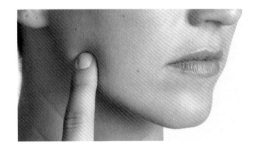

Helps with these conditions

- toothache in the lower jaw
- temporomandibular joint (TMJ) pain
- gum disease
- deviation of the mouth after a stroke

Stomach 7 (ST-7 / Xiaguan)

This point is located on the jaw.

1 To locate the point, look at your face in a mirror.

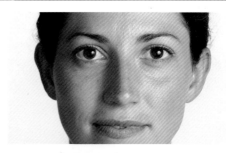

2 Locate the top of the cheekbone and slide an index finger along the outer edge of it toward the ear until it runs into the joint of the jaw. To test that the finger is at the joint, open the mouth wide — it should feel as though the jawbone is pushing the finger out of the depression.

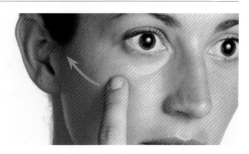

3 The fingertip should be in a depression about one thumb's width from the tragus, the small flap of cartilage at the front of the ear.

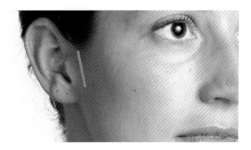

4 The direct center of this depression is where you will find the point.

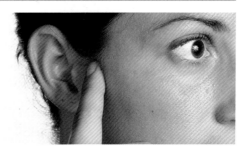

Helps with these conditions

- skin blemishes (acne)
- deafness, tinnitus, ear pain
- toothache of the upper jaw
- muscle spasms of the face
- facial nerve pain (trigeminal neuralgia)

Stomach 8 (ST-8 / Touwei)

This point is located on the head at the upper corners of the face, just inside the hairline.

1. To locate the point, look at your face in a mirror. With the tip of the index finger, find the outer end of the eyebrow.

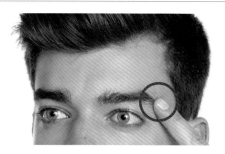

2. Slide the index finger straight up from the inner temple (the part of the temple closest to the end of the eyebrow) until the finger is about four fingers' width above the eyebrow.

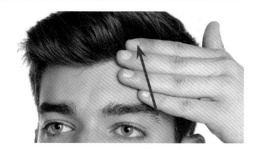

3. Next, note the divot at the hairline, then extend the index finger into the hairline about another half an inch (1 cm) beyond the divot to the slight depression further back on the head.

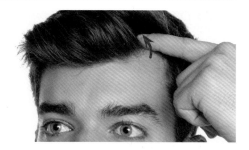

4. Where the finger lands on the center of this depression is where you will find the point.

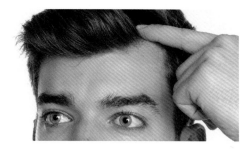

Helps with these conditions

- hair loss (alopecia)
- frontal headache
- splitting headache
- excessive eye tearing, especially with outdoor activity
- one-sided facial paralysis

Stomach 25 (ST-25 / Tianshu)

This point is located on the abdomen, at the level of the belly button, or umbilicus.

1 To locate the point, lie down and expose the lower abdomen. Locate the belly button. Place three fingers vertically (fingertips pointing down) against the lower abdomen, measured from the belly button, so that the edge of the index finger is against the outer edge of the belly button.

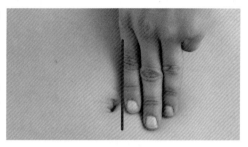

2 Where the third finger ends up on the abdomen, mark an imaginary vertical line. Slide the tip of the index finger along an imaginary horizontal line to the point where the two lines intersect. Where there is a slight depression you will find the point. Note the point.

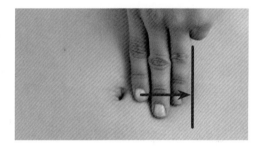

3 Next, locate the point on the opposite side of the abdomen.

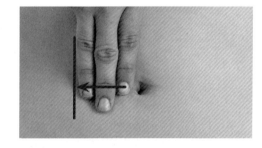

4 Using the index fingers, press both points at the same time.

✳ **Warning:** Avoid during pregnancy — can cause contractions. **Warning:** Avoid during pregnancy — may cause too much pressure on the baby.

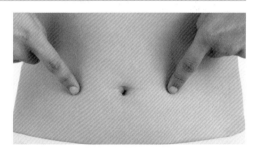

Helps with these conditions

- constipation
- all intestinal imbalances

Stomach 36 (ST-36 / Zusanli)

This point is located on the lower leg, one hand's width down from the knee crease, and one thumb's width to the right of the shinbone.

1 To locate the point, extend your leg while seated on a bed or floor.

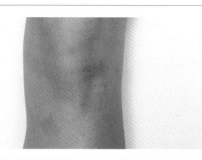

2 Place your left hand on your right lower leg (shin) so that the index finger bumps up against the kneecap (patella). Where your pinky finger falls is the horizontal location line where you will find the point. Note the line and remove your left hand from your shin.

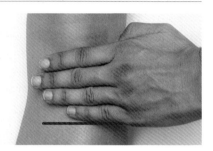

3 Next, place your right thumb vertically next to the shinbone so that the left edge of your thumb presses against the shinbone, and the widest part of your thumb falls across the horizontal line you just located. The right side of your thumb defines the vertical location line. Note this line.

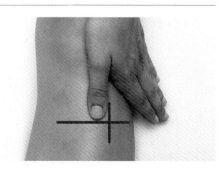

4 Where these two location lines intersect is where you will find the point.

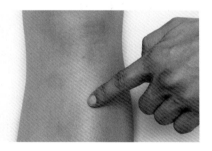

Helps with these conditions

- bloating, intestinal imbalances
- constipation and diarrhea
- ulcer
- ringing in the ears (tinnitus)
- dizziness
- chills and fever

Stomach 40 (ST-40 / Fenglong)

This point is located on the lower leg.

1 To locate the point, sit in a chair with both feet flat on the ground and the knees bent. Find the lower edge of the kneecap (patella). This is the upper location line. Note the line.

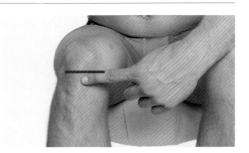

2 Next, locate the front ankle crease. To find this line, with the index finger held horizontally, slide it from the toes up the foot until it runs into the ankle, right before the 90-degree bend created by the lower leg. This is the lower location line.

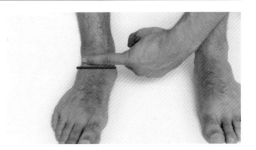

3 Next, slide the index finger down from the upper location line, along the shinbone (tibia) to find the midpoint between these two lines — it should be around two-hands width down from the upper location line.

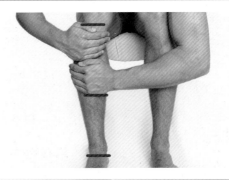

4 Slide the index finger to the outer side of the lower leg along a horizontal line two fingers' width. This is where you will find the point.

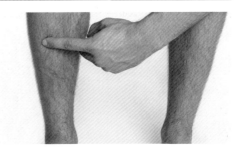

Helps with these conditions

- phlegm
- cough
- wheezing
- pain and fullness in the chest and throat
- loss of voice
- bipolar disorder

Spleen 4 (SP-4 / Gongsun)

This point is located on the inner side of the foot.

1 To locate the point, sit in a chair and cross one ankle over the opposite knee to allow easy access to the foot. Locate the large protruding bone at the first joint of the big toe.

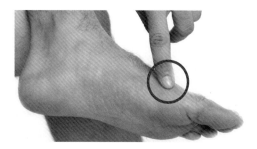

2 With an index finger, roll off the large bone diagonally, in the direction of the bottom of the foot until you feel the first long thin metatarsal bone.

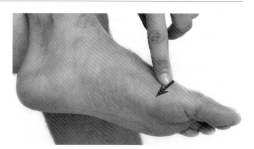

3 Next, slide the finger along the metatarsal bone toward the ankle. You should feel the large tendon on the bottom of the foot on the other side of your finger.

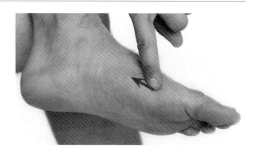

4 Continue to slide the index finger along the first metatarsal bone. Where it lands on a depression between the tendon of the foot and the upper end of the first metatarsal bone is where you will find the point.

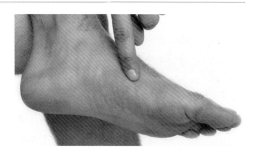

Helps with these conditions

- indigestion, especially with pain or cold sensation in the gastrointestinal tract (GI)
- bloating
- gurgling in the GI
- lack of appetite

Spleen 6 (SP-6 / Sanyinjiao)

This point is located on the lower leg.

1 To locate the point, sit in a chair and cross one ankle over the opposite knee to allow easy access to the lower leg. Locate the inner ankle bone.

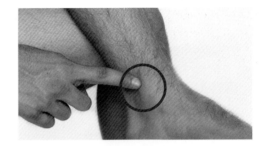

2 Next, place four fingers across the lower leg, with the outer edge of the pinky finger pressing against the ankle bone. Note this line.

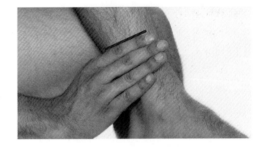

3 Locate the inner back edge of the shinbone (tibia).

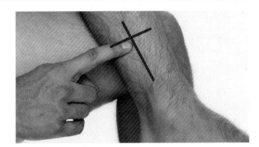

4 Where these two location lines intersect is where you will find the point.

✳ Warning: Avoid during pregnancy — can cause contractions.

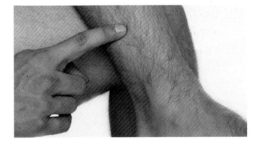

Helps with these conditions

- allergies
- all female and male reproductive imbalances
- any digestive issues

- diabetes
- edema
- fungal infections
- bedwetting (nocturnal enuresis)

Spleen 8 (SP-8 / Diji)

This point is located on the inner lower leg.

① To locate the point, find the knee crease at the back of the leg, on the inner side.

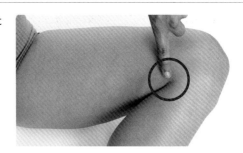

② Place four fingers of one hand horizontally against the inner lower leg so that the pinky finger lines up with the back knee crease.

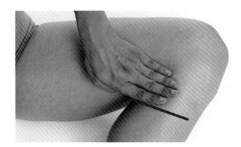

③ Next, place three fingers of the other hand immediately below the four fingers already on the lower leg so that seven fingers line up below the knee crease. Where the lower edge of the lowest finger intersects the back edge of the shinbone is where you will find the point.

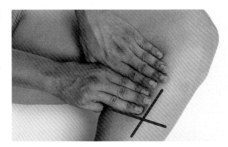

④ To find it, remove the first hand and palpate for the slight depression.

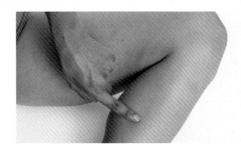

Helps with these conditions

- anemia
- irregular menstruation
- painful menstruation, especially acute onset

Spleen 10 (SP-10 / Xuehai)

This point is located on the inner leg just above the knee.

1 To locate the point, extend your legs while seated on a bed or floor.

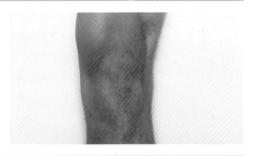

2 Place the index and middle fingers of one hand horizontally across the leg above the knee, so that the lower edge of the middle finger sits on the upper margin of the kneecap. The second joint of both fingers should be right above the center of the kneecap.

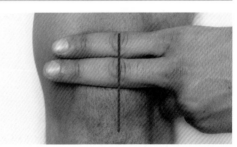

3 Next, slide the index finger toward the inner thigh about an inch (2.5 cm), so that the tip of the index finger lands about 1 inch further down the curve of the inner thigh than it was.

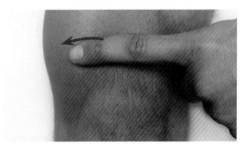

4 Where the tip of the index finger lands on a slight depression is where you will find the point.

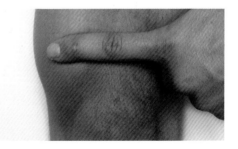

Helps with these conditions

- bruising and hematoma
- blood stasis
- blood deficiency
- excess bleeding
- varicose veins, hemorrhoids (varicosities)
- anemia in postpartum
- hot and itching conditions of the skin

Heart 7 (Ht-7 / Shenmen)

This point is located on the forearm, at the wrist crease.

1 To locate the point, rest the hand on a comfortable surface, palm side facing up.

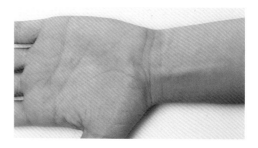

2 Locate the wrist crease by slightly bending the hand up. Relax the hand.

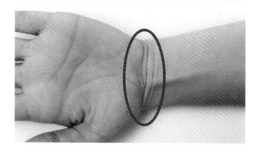

3 Next, slide the tip of the index finger along the wrist crease toward the small bone of the wrist located directly beneath the pinky finger.

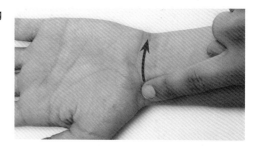

4 Where the wrist crease and the wrist bone meet is where you will find the point.

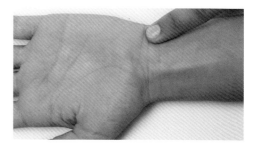

Helps with these conditions

- acute cold and flu symptoms, especially phlegm
- Raynaud syndrome
- headache due to stiff neck
- all postpartum imbalances
- depression

Small Intestine 1 (SI-1 / Shaoze)

This point is located on the pinky finger, near the nail.

1 To locate the point, place the hand on a flat surface, palm side down. Find the bottom of the nail on the pinky finger.

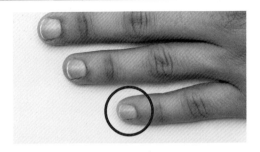

2 Note a location line at the bottom of the nail.

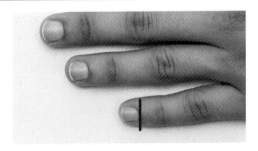

3 Next, note a line along the outer side of the nail.

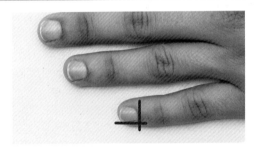

4 Where these two lines intersect is where you will find the point.

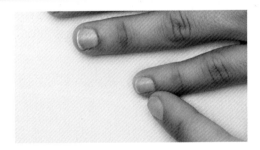

Helps with these conditions

- mastitis
- breast distention
- breast congestion
- clogged milk ducts

Small Intestine 3 (SI-3 / Houxi)

This point is located on the outer side of the hand.

1 To locate the point, slide the tip of the index finger along the pinky finger toward the wrist.

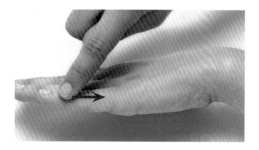

2 Slide the tip of the finger over the first joint of the pinky finger and onto a depression on the outer side of the hand.

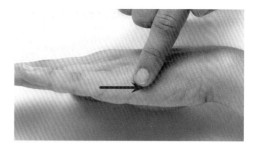

3 The depression lies between the pad on the outer edge of the palm (the hypothenar eminence) and the long bone along the side of the hand (the metacarpal of the pinky finger).

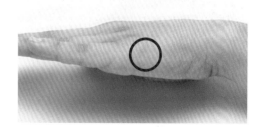

4 Where the finger lands on the center of this depression is where you will find the point.

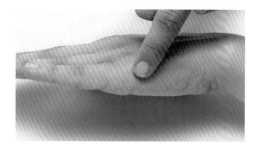

Helps with these conditions

- arthritis
- neck spasm, stiff neck (torticollis)
- shaking or trembling limbs
- conditions related to the sensory organs

Bladder 1 (BL-1 / Jingming)

This point is located on the face, in between the nose and the inner corner of the eye (inner canthus), and slightly above it.

1 To locate the point, look at your face in a mirror.

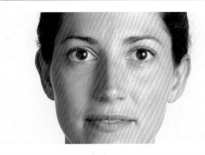

2 Locate the inner canthus, the area where the two eyelids come together, close to the nose.

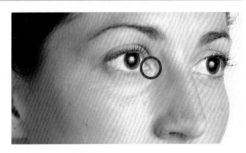

3 Next, gently place an index finger over the inner eyelid until the tip of the finger is resting in the inner canthus.

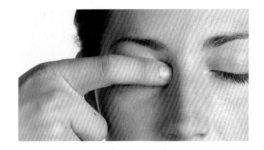

4 Very gently apply pressure to the eyeball while rolling the tip of the finger over it until the fingertip rolls over the innermost edge of the bone of the eye socket. Where the finger falls into the gap between the eyeball and the bone of the eye socket is where you will find the point. This point is held, not pressed.

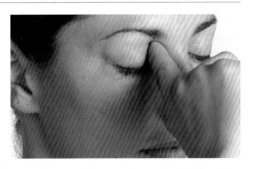

Helps with these conditions

- pinkeye (conjunctivitis) — to avoid spreading, treat the opposite eye
- excessive tearing
- most conditions of the eyes: dry, bloodshot, irritated, itching

Bladder 2 (BL-2 / Zanzhu)

This point is located on the face, at the inner edge of the eyebrow.

1 To locate the point, look at your face in a mirror.

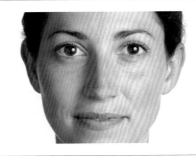

2 Locate the inner edge of the eyebrow.

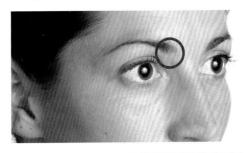

3 Next, locate the inner canthus of the eye, the area where the two eyelids come together, close to the nose.

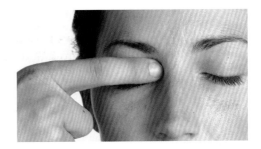

4 Slide the tip of the index finger from the hollow at the inner canthus up in the direction of the inner end of the eyebrow. Where the finger lands on a slight dip at the inner eyebrow is where you will find the point.

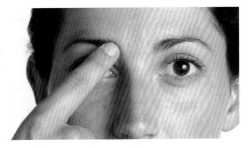

Helps with these conditions

- allergies
- frontal headache
- blurred vision
- eyelid twitching
- rectal prolapse (protrusion)

Bladder 40 (BL-40 / Weizhong)

This point is located on the lower leg, on the back of the knee.

1 To locate the point, sit in a chair with both feet flat on the ground and the knees bent. Locate the tendon that defines the outside border of the back of the knee.

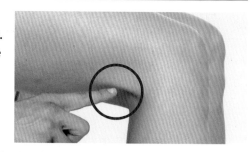

2 Next, locate the other tendons that define the inner border of the back of the knee. Both of these tendons can easily be felt when the knee is bent, by palpating with fingers behind the knee while tensing the muscles of the upper leg.

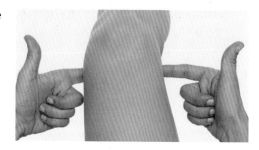

3 Next, with your index finger, reach into the soft tissue behind the knee at the level of the back knee crease.

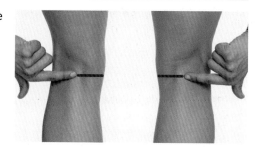

4 Where the finger lands on a depression at the center point midway between the two tendons is where you will find the point.

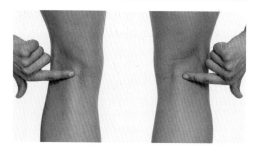

Helps with these conditions

- chronic or acute low back pain or stiffness
- chronic or acute knee pain or stiffness
- tendon stiffness
- all back pain

Bladder 67 (BL-67 / Zhiyin)

This point is located on the outer edge of the pinky toe.

1 To locate the point, sit in a chair and cross one ankle over the opposite knee to allow easy access to the foot.

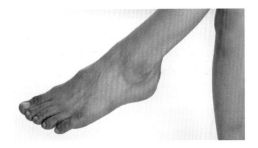

2 Locate the outer edge of the toenail on the pinky toe and note this line.

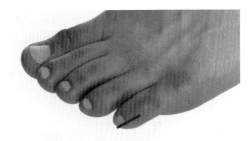

3 Next, locate the base of the toenail and note this line.

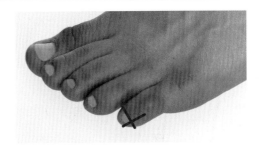

4 Where these two location lines intersect is where you will find the point.

✳ **Warning:** Avoid during pregnancy — can cause contractions.

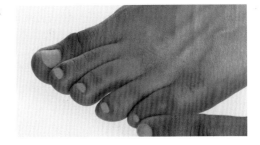

Helps with these conditions

- heat in the head
- nasal congestion
- nosebleed
- heaviness in the head
- heat in the feet

Kidney 1 (KI-1 / Yongquan)

This point is located on the bottom of the foot.

1 To locate the point, sit in a chair or on a flat surface.

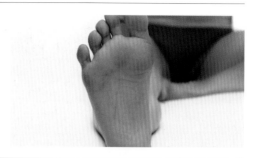

2 Locate the midline at the bottom of the foot.

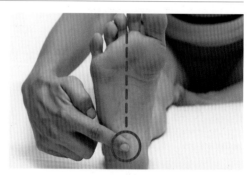

3 Next, slide your index finger along the midline of the sole of the foot toward the toes until it lands on the large depression just before the ball of the foot.

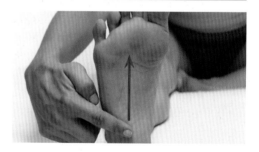

4 Where the finger lands on this depression is where you will find the point.

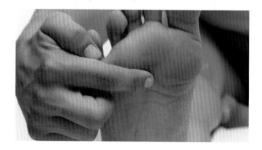

Helps with these conditions

- plantar fasciitis
- anxiety
- insomnia
- constipation (lack of movement in the lower abdomen)
- dizziness
- difficulty urinating

Kidney 3 (KI-3 / Taixi)

This point is located on the inner ankle.

1 To locate the point, sit in a chair and cross one ankle over the opposite knee to allow easy access to the ankle.

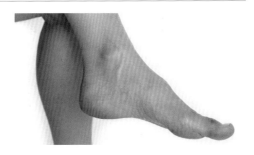

2 Locate the highest point of the inner ankle bone.

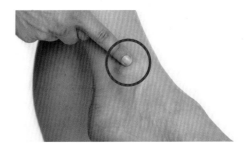

3 Next, from there, slide the tip of the index finger back toward the Achilles tendon, the large tendon that connects the calf to the foot, until the finger lands on a depression.

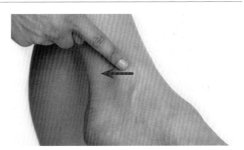

4 Where the finger lands on the center of this depression is where you will find the point.

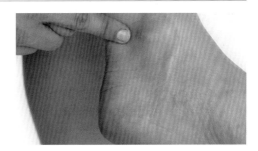

Helps with these conditions

- chronic/adrenal fatigue
- asthma
- seminal emissions
- excessive urination
- bedwetting, urinary incontinence
- ringing in the ears (tinnitus)
- dizziness
- heat in the head
- cold at the extremities
- nosebleed and cough

Kidney 6 (KI-6 / Zhaohai)

This point is located on the inner foot below the inner ankle bone.

1 To locate the point, sit in a chair and cross one ankle over the opposite knee to allow easy access to the ankle.

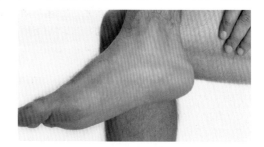

2 Locate your inner ankle bone.

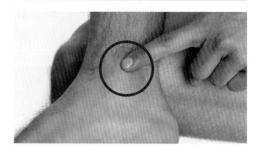

3 Next, from there, slide the tip of the index finger from the ankle bone down, until it drops into a depression located about one thumb's width below the bone.

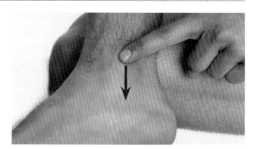

4 Where the finger lands on this depression is where you will find the point.

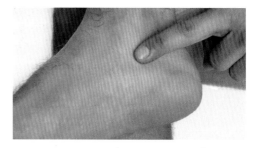

Helps with these conditions

- chronic fatigue
- hot flashes
- sore throat
- incontinence
- diarrhea
- menopausal symptoms
- leukorrhea (vaginal discharge)
- scanty menstruation

Kidney 9 (KI-9 / Zhubin)

This point is located on the inner part of the lower leg.

1 To locate the point, sit in a chair and cross one ankle over the opposite knee to allow easy access to the lower leg.

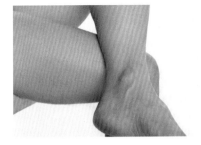

2 Locate the highest point of the inner ankle bone.

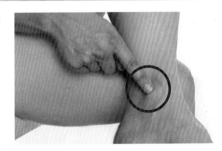

3 Next, measure seven fingers' width above the inner ankle bone. Note the horizontal line. The point is located one thumb's width from the inner edge of the shinbone (tibia) toward the calf.

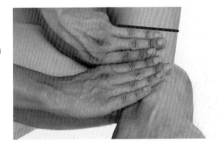

4 With the lower leg crossed and relaxed over the other leg, you will find the point approximately midway between the shin and the calf.

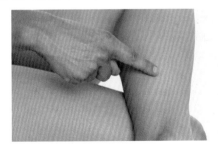

Helps with these conditions

- feeling disconnected
- bipolar disorder
- anxiety
- insomnia
- lack of purpose
- heat in the upper body
- cold in the lower body

Pericardium 6 (PC-6 / Neiguan)

This point is located on the inner forearm close to the wrist.

1. To locate the point, rest the arm on a comfortable surface, palm side facing up.

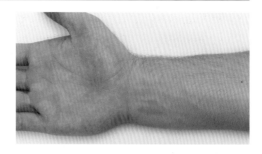

2. Place two middle fingers from your left hand on your right forearm so that the middle finger lays facedown over the wrist crease. Where the index finger falls is the horizontal location line. Note the line and remove your left hand from your forearm.

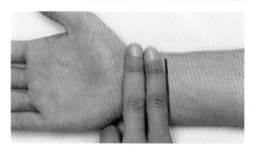

3. Next, locate the tendon in the center of the forearm by bending your hand at the wrist so that the palm is moving up, toward the elbow.

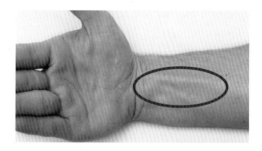

4. Where the horizontal location line intersects the tendon is where you will find the point. Bring your hand back down before pressing the point.

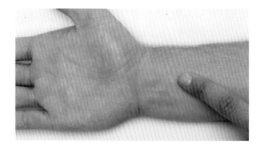

Helps with these conditions

- addiction
- chest pain (angina pectoris)
- nausea and vomiting
- morning sickness

- anxiety
- insomnia
- conditions of the chest

Pericardium 7 (PC-7 / Daling)

This point is located on the inner forearm, on the wrist crease.

1 To locate the point, rest the hand on a comfortable surface, palm side facing up. Locate the wrist crease by slightly bending the hand up. Relax the hand.

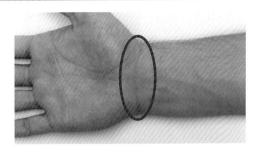

2 Next, locate the tendon at the center of the wrist.

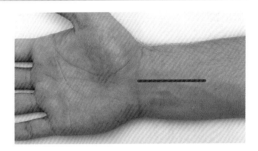

3 Tensing all fingers will engage the tendon, making it easier to find.

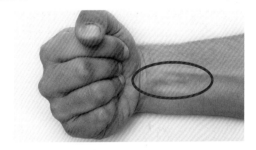

4 Where the wrist crease and the tendon intersect is where you will find the point.

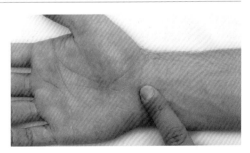

Helps with these conditions

- carpal tunnel syndrome
- heart pain
- palpitations

- shortness of breath
- fullness or pain in the chest

Triple Warmer 3 (TW-3 / Zhongzhu)

This point is located on the back side of the hand.

1 To locate the point, find the webbing between the fourth (ring) and fifth (pinky) fingers.

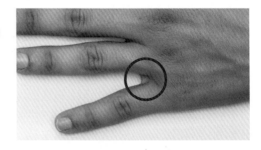

2 With the opposite hand, slide the tip of the index finger from the webbing between the fourth and fifth finger toward the wrist, sliding just over the bones of the first joint between the fingers and the hand and into the first depression.

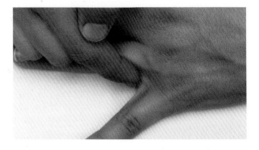

3 The finger's tip should be about two fingers' width from the end of the webbing between the two fingers.

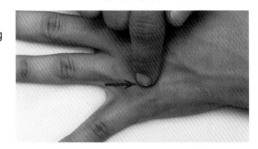

4 Where the finger lands on this first depression is where you will find the point.

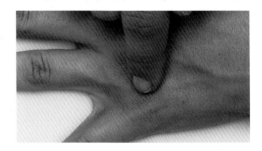

Helps with these conditions

- ringing in the ears (tinnitus), especially sudden onset
- earache, especially due to exposure to cold wind
- deafness
- one-sided headache

Triple Warmer 14 (TW-14 / Jianliao)

This point is located on the back shoulder, at the shoulder joint.

1 To locate the point, stand in front of a mirror. Bend the arm 90 degrees and raise the elbow until it is level with the shoulder.

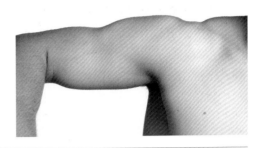

2 This will cause two depressions to appear next to each other at the top of the shoulder. If they are not obvious, palpate for them just above the deltoid muscle at the top of the arm.

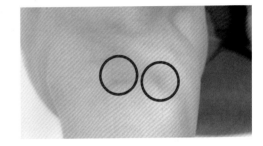

3 Next, use the index finger from the opposite hand to find the depression at the back of the shoulder.

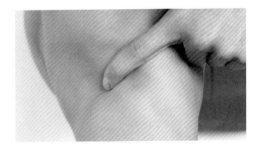

4 Where the finger lands on the depression closest to the back is where you will find the point. Be sure to relax the arm before pressing the point.

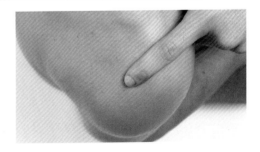

Helps with these conditions

- frozen shoulder (adhesive capsulitis), especially at the back of the shoulder
- numbness or pain of the shoulder or arm

Gallbladder 20 (GB-20 / Fengchi)

This point is located on the back of the head.

1 To locate the point, find the bony prominence at the back of the head, about one hand's width above the back hairline.

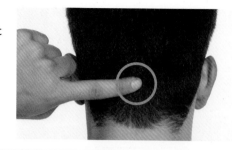

2 Slide the tip of the index finger over this prominence until it lands on a depression.

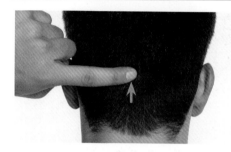

3 Next, move the index finger to the outer side along the bony ridge about three fingers' width, until it hits a fleshy mound.

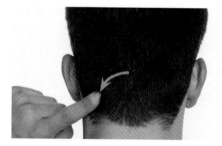

4 Where the finger lands in the center of this mound is where you will find the point.

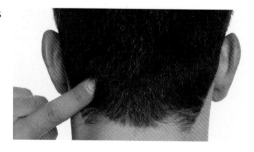

Helps with these conditions

- insomnia
- all conditions on the face
- temporal headache

- one-sided headache
- stiffness and rigidity of the neck
- excessive tearing, especially due to wind (lacrimation)

Gallbladder 30 (GB-30 / Huantiao)

This point is located on the buttocks.

1 To locate the point, stand in a relaxed position.

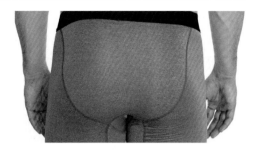

2 With your fingers, find the large depression at the center of one of the buttock cheeks.

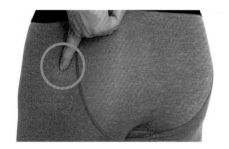

3 This point falls on a line drawn from the tip of the tailbone (coccyx) to the hip socket.

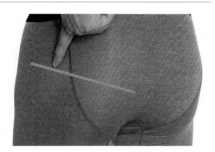

4 Where the finger lands on the center of this depression is where you will find the point.

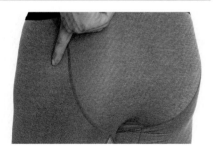

Helps with these conditions

- sciatica
- pain in the hip or buttock
- lumbar pain
- pain or numbness in the leg
- atrophy of the limbs

Gallbladder 34 (GB-34 / Yanglingquan)

This point is located on the lower leg, near the knee.

1. To locate the point, sit in a chair with both feet flat on the ground and the knees bent.

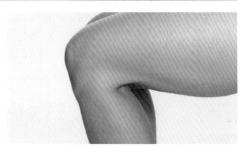

2. With your fingers, locate the fibula bone, found toward the outside of the leg, next to the larger shinbone (tibia).

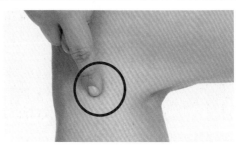

3. Next, slide the finger down from the knee until it lands on a large depression just under the head of the fibula. The head of the fibula connects with the knee, so the location of this point is quite close to the knee.

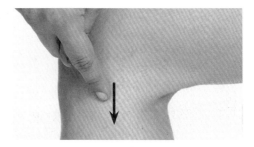

4. Where your finger lands, about three fingers' width below the level of the back knee crease, is where you will find the point.

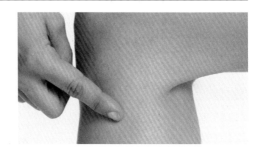

Helps with these conditions

- disorders of the sinews, tendons, ligaments and connective tissue
- most nerve disorders
- stiffness in the limbs (especially knees)
- atrophy of the limbs
- facial nerve pain (trigeminal neuralgia); sciatica

Gallbladder 43 (GB-43 / Xiaxi)

This point is located on the foot.

1 To locate the point, sit in a chair and cross the ankle over the opposite knee to allow easy access to the foot.

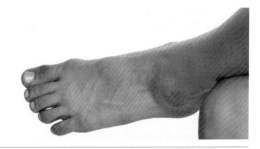

2 Locate the toe crease between the fourth and fifth toes.

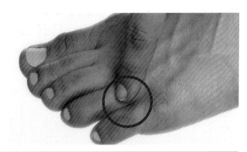

3 Next, slide your finger in the direction of the ankle along the toe crease.

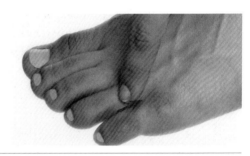

4 Where the tip of the finger slides up just barely out of the toe crease is where you will find the point.

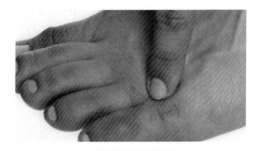

Helps with these conditions

- throbbing in the head upon standing
- hypertension
- red eyes
- fullness of the chest

Liver 3 (LR-3 / Taichong)

This point is located on the top of the foot.

1 To locate the point, sit in a chair and cross one ankle over the opposite knee to allow easy access to the foot.

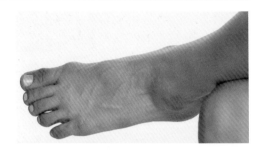

2 Locate the webbing between the big and second toes.

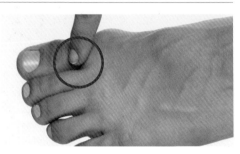

3 Next, slide the tip of the index finger along the valley between the tendons of these two toes until it lands on a depression, about one thumb's width from the end of the toe crease. Make sure the tip of the finger is centered between the tendons of the big toe and the second toe.

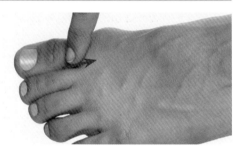

4 Where the finger lands on the center of this depression is where you will find the point.

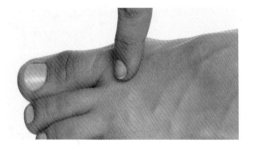

Helps with these conditions

- hepatitis
- spasmodic cough
- abdominal pain
- genital pain
- difficulty arising upon waking
- dizziness
- shortness of breath
- irregular menstruation

Liver 8 (LR-8 / Ququan)

This point is located on the leg, close to the inner knee.

1 To locate the point, extend the leg and find the bottom edge of the kneecap (patella).

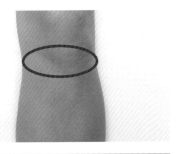

2 Lay four fingers across the kneecap on the opposite leg so that the outer edge of the pinky finger sits at the bottom of the kneecap. The index finger should be resting on a line that extends through the fleshy tissue on the inner leg.

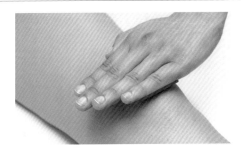

3 Next, slide the tip of the index finger about an inch down the curve of the inner thigh until it is on the highest point of this fleshy area.

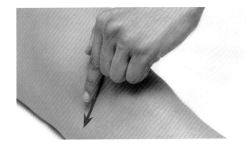

4 Where the tip of the finger rests on this highest point is where you will find the point.

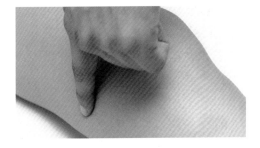

Helps with these conditions

- anxiety manifesting as mania
- impotence
- itching of the genitals
- vaginal discharge (leukorrhea)
- involuntary ejaculation (spermatorrhea)

Conception Vessel 4 (CV-4 / Guanyuan)

This point is located on the lower abdomen.

1 To locate the point, stand in front of a mirror. Expose the lower abdomen.

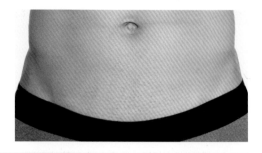

2 Locate the belly button (umbilicus). Place a finger on it.

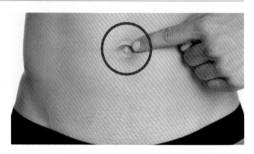

3 Next, slide the finger down about four fingers' width.

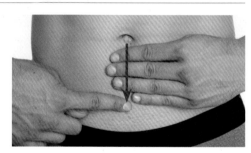

4 Where the finger lands on the swell of tissue just under the belly button is where you will find the point.

✳ **Warning:** Avoid during pregnancy — may cause too much pressure on the baby.

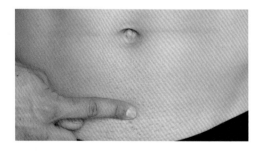

Helps with these conditions

- exhaustion
- weakness
- low-back pain
- deficiency conditions of all kinds

- infertility
- urinary incontinence
- shrinking/wasting of the limbs (muscle atrophy)

Conception Vessel 10 (CV-10 / Xiawan)

This point is located on the abdomen.

1. To locate the point, stand in front of a mirror. Expose the abdomen.

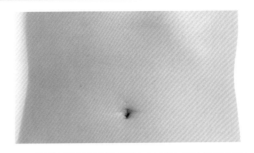

2. Locate the belly button (umbilicus). Place a finger on it.

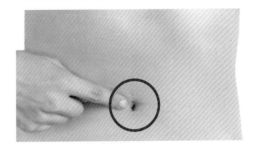

3. Next, slide the tip of the index finger three fingers' width up from the belly button.

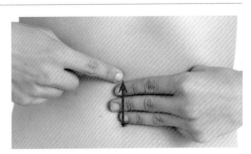

4. Where the finger lands on a depression is where you will find the point.

   ✴ **Warning:** Avoid during pregnancy — may cause too much pressure on the baby.

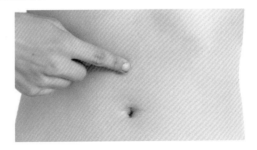

Helps with these conditions

- indigestion
- food stagnation
- undigested food in the stool
- nausea or vomiting, especially after eating

Conception Vessel 12 (CV-12 / Zhongwan)

This point is located on the abdomen.

1 To locate the point, stand in front of a mirror. Expose the abdomen.

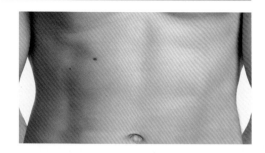

2 Slide the index finger to locate the bottom of the xiphoid process, the lower end of the breastbone (sternum). If the xiphoid itself cannot be located, find the point where the ribs join the low end of the breastbone as a reference point.

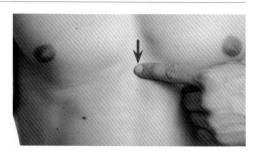

3 Next, locate the belly button (umbilicus).

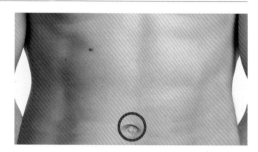

4 The midway point between these two structures, about six fingers' width down from the sternum or up from the belly button, is where you will find the point.

✳ Warning: Avoid during pregnancy — may cause too much pressure on the baby.

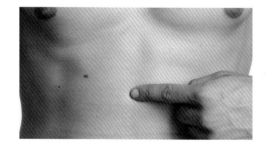

Helps with these conditions

- all digestive conditions
- diarrhea
- heartburn, acid reflux (gastroesophageal reflux disease, or GERD)
- lack of appetite
- the habit of eating to relieve stress
- easily feeling full
- vomiting

Conception Vessel 22 (CV-22 / Tiantu)

This point is located on the lower neck.

1 To locate the point, stand in front of a mirror.

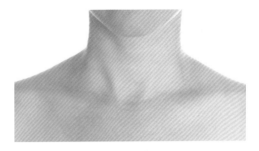

2 Slide the index finger over the breastbone (sternum) to find the notch in the center of the top of this bone.

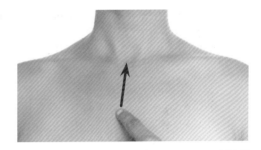

3 The point is actually located behind the bone, so it is best pressed by gently rolling the finger up and over the breastbone, into the hollow behind it.

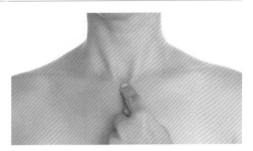

4 Be careful not to apply pressure to the Adam's apple (hyoid bone), which is located just above this point.

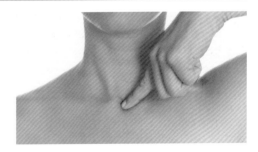

Helps with these conditions

- cough with thin, colorless secretions
- esophageal constriction
- persistent tickle in the throat
- loss of voice
- dry throat
- thyroid imbalance

Conception Vessel 23 (CV-23 / Lianquan)

This point is located on the upper neck, just under the chin.

1 To locate the point, stand in front of a mirror.

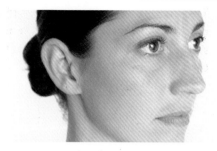

2 Locate the juncture where the neck and the chin come together at the center of the neck.

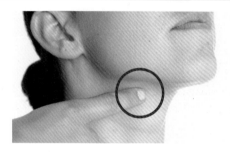

3 It is easiest to locate this point when the head is at a neutral position, facing forward, chin slightly raised. When the point is pressed, it will be felt at the back of the tongue.

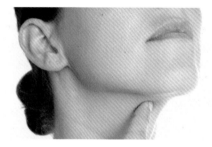

4 Next, press the point gently with the index finger approximately at a 45-degree angle, in order to avoid closing the airways (trachea). Avoid putting pressure on the Adam's apple (hyoid bone), which is located just below this point.

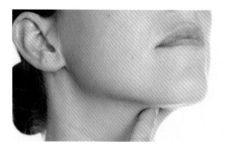

Helps with these conditions

- mouth sores
- bad breath (halitosis)
- bleeding gums
- excessive or deficient salivation
- vomiting foam

Governing Vessel 20 (GV-20 / Baihui)

This point is located on the top of the head.

1 To locate the point, stand in front of a mirror. Place both index fingers along the side of the face where the ear attaches to the face.

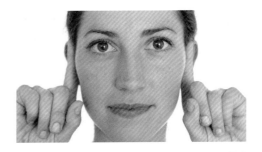

2 Next, follow an imaginary line that runs from the front of each ear to the top of the head.

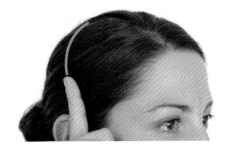

3 Where these two lines intersect at the top of the head, approximately eight fingers' width from the front hairline, is where you will find the point.

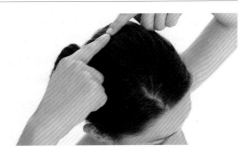

4 For some people, this point may be slightly forward or behind — it is usually tender or sensitive, so it is easily located by a sensation of tenderness.

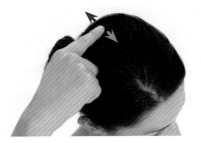

Helps with these conditions

- pain at the top of the head
- dizziness upon standing
- vertigo and light-headedness
- uterine or rectal prolapse
- poor memory
- foggy brain

Yintang

This point is located on the face, between the eyebrows.

1 To locate the point, stand in front of a mirror.

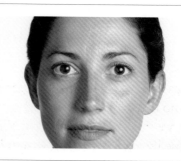

2 Locate the area between the eyebrows. There may be a raised area or it may be flat.

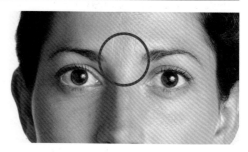

3 Next, find the horizontal location line that marks the highest point of the brows. Note this line. Find the groove that marks the bottom of the square between the brows. Note this groove.

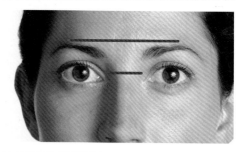

4 At the very center of the square defined by the horizontal location line and the groove is where you will find the point. For many people, the point is equidistant from the inner ends of the eyebrows and the groove that marks the bottom of the square between the brows.

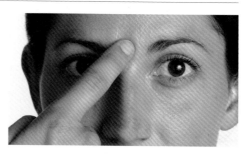

Helps with these conditions

- fright
- insomnia
- restlessness
- agitation

Acknowledgments

It has been said in many different ways, but no matter how we phrase it, it is true that we stand on the shoulders of those whose lives inform our understanding. I have been utterly shaped by the teachings of my mentor, Dr. Heiner Fruehauf. Heiner taught his students to look to the classics of Chinese thought for insight into nature, including human nature. A deep study of these classics — texts such as *Huangdi Neijing Suwen, Daode Jing, Zhuangzi* and many others — allowed me to really grasp the foundational ideas of Chinese medicine, which is rooted in the observable patterns of nature. As Heiner often reminded us, the ideas found in Chinese medicine are applicable to everything, because they are universal principles. I am forever grateful to Heiner for helping me to unlearn the modern way of viewing reality, allowing me to be in profound relationship with the Everything. If I had not first learned to see through the overcultural projection that severs us from the natural wisdom that surrounds us, I am sure my learning would have been far less deep and impactful.

I will always be indebted to Dr. Brandt Stickley, who further shifted my perspective through an application of the Chinese medical concepts to psychology. The simple sophistication of Dr. Leon Hammer's work, as received from Brandt, continues to support me when addressing the mental, emotional and spiritual aspects of my patients.

As I navigate the last steps of working toward a PhD in psychology, I want to acknowledge the incredible impact of another teacher, Ishtar Kramer. Ishtar lives what she teaches, and her vulnerability and honesty have radically shifted how I understand my own heart. Most of us have had the joy of learning from someone whose teachings stay with us always, and I am very clear that Ishtar's understanding of our relationship with our own self is foundational to my experience of being authentically alive.

As I become a more authentic person, my relationships with my loved ones have become so beautiful. My mom and I now love each other fully and without judgment. My mother, Daphne Clausen, is one of the greatest blessings in my life, and I am very grateful for her.

Finally, I credit my partner, Max, with bringing me back to life at a time when I was completely checked out and simply waiting around for my life to end. When I had given up on myself, and honestly, humanity in general, Max entered my life like a beam of light straight from the One. I simply cannot imagine my life without them, nor are there words adequate to describe the depth of my gratitude for their presence. Love you forever, my heart.

Resources

Interested in learning more? If this little book has sparked an interest in learning more about the topics discussed, consider the resources listed below.

CHINESE MEDICINE

Chinese Medicine: The Web That Has No Weaver, by Ted Kaptchuk

This book is an excellent introduction to the basic concepts, applications, and modalities of Chinese medicine. Approachable and interesting, it is a great place to start expanding your understanding of this ancient system.

Between Heaven and Earth: A Guide to Chinese Medicine, by Harriet Beinfield and Efrem Korngold

Another classic introduction to the concepts, this book has been enjoyed by thousands interested in learning more about Chinese medicine. For many, this was the book that started them on their journey to becoming a practitioner, but it is comprehensible for the armchair learner as well.

The Yellow Emperor's Classic of Medicine, by Maoshing Ni.

Ni is credited as the translator, but I find this to be more of an interpretation of the original. This book is highly readable and will definitely give the reader a feel for the classical text of Chinese medicine, *Huangdi NeiJing Suwen.*

CHINESE PHILOSOPHY

Daode Jing

There are literally millions of translations of this classic of Daoism, one of the fundamental philosophies that informs Chinese medicine. It is the fourth-most translated book of all time.

Some of my favorite translations are listed here:

Lao Tzu: Tao Te Ching: A Book about the Way and the Power of the Way, by Laozi, translated by Ursula K. Le Guin

Ursula K. Le Guin is my favorite author; her perspective is always unique and informative.

Lao-tzu's Taoteching, translated by Red Pine

One of the world's leading translators of Chinese texts, Red Pine's translation is both scholarly and approachable.

Tao Te Ching, by Lao Tzu (Author), Gia-Fu Feng (Translator), Jane English (Translator)

I like this one because the translators have removed some of the gendered language that is not found in the original Chinese, making it truer to the classical version.

ANATOMY

Trail Guide to the Body: How to Locate Muscles, Bones and More, 5th Edition, by Andrew Biel

If you found the locating the acupoints to be interesting, and would like to learn more about anatomy, this guide is by far the easiest, most useful guide I have found. I use this when teaching palpation to my Chinese medicine students!

Library and Archives Canada Cataloguing in Publication

Title: The beginner's guide to acupressure : DIY steps for self-care / Karin Parramore, LAc, CH.
Other titles: Essential step-by-step guide to acupressure with aromatherapy
Names: Parramore, Karin, 1964- author.
Description: Previously published under title: The essential step-by-step guide to acupressure with aromatherapy : relief for 64 common health conditions. | Includes index.
Identifiers: Canadiana 20240338650 | ISBN 9780778807223 (softcover)
Subjects: LCSH: Acupressure.
Classification: LCC RM723.A27 P37 2024 | DDC 615.8/222—dc23

INDEX